Janet Carolina Negrón Espadas
Aurora Sierra Canto

Nursing and Occupational Health

Janet Carolina Negrón Espadas
Aurora Sierra Canto

Nursing and Occupational Health

Nursing Challenges

Imprint

Any brand names and product names mentioned in this book are subject to trademark, brand or patent protection and are trademarks or registered trademarks of their respective holders. The use of brand names, product names, common names, trade names, product descriptions etc. even without a particular marking in this work is in no way to be construed to mean that such names may be regarded as unrestricted in respect of trademark and brand protection legislation and could thus be used by anyone.

Cover image: www.ingimage.com

This book is a translation from the original published under ISBN 978-620-2-09943-1.

Publisher:
Sciencia Scripts
is a trademark of
Dodo Books Indian Ocean Ltd. and OmniScriptum S.R.L publishing group

120 High Road, East Finchley, London, N2 9ED, United Kingdom
Str. Armeneasca 28/1, office 1, Chisinau MD-2012, Republic of Moldova, Europe
Printed at: see last page
ISBN: 978-620-5-82812-0

Introduction

The International Labour Organisation establishes the principle of protection for workers against illness in general or occupational diseases and accidents resulting from their work. Therefore, occupational health is an issue of great relevance as it is the element that impacts on workers in taking advantage of opportunities to develop, improve their social relations and enhance their self-esteem within an organisation. It also enables health professionals to manage strategies to reduce absenteeism, improve the working environment, motivation and reduce risks in the workplace.

In this respect, according to global estimates, the economic costs are mainly caused by illness or death arising from the workplace. This affects the worker, families, companies and the country, which can result in early retirement, loss of qualified personnel, absenteeism and high insurance premiums, but these tragedies can be avoided by adopting rational methods of prevention, reporting and timely inspection.

Within the framework of the above considerations, it is clear that the more disease prevention, the better the chances of improving health and maintaining it in optimal conditions for the population and therefore for the system, which is a necessary premise in occupational health. Thus, the structure of the health system and primary health care are responsible for maintaining the state of well-being.

This book aims to introduce the reader to current occupational health issues from the health, social, ethical and legal perspectives.

The book is made up of two sections, the first on Nursing and Occupational Health and the second on two topics relevant to women in the work context, i.e. Gender-Based Violence and Breastfeeding.

The first section, entitled Nursing and Occupational Health, is made up of five chapters. Throughout this section, the background to the practice of nursing in health and the current challenges that frame the path to follow are addressed, based on the historical, cultural, economic and technological facts that influence professional practice. Taking up what was analysed in the previous section but with a competent approach to nursing, as there is no doubt that among the challenges faced by health personnel are the changes in health policy, the introduction of innovations in hospitals, in medical technology, the reorientation of diagnosis-oriented medicine towards preventive practices and thus the strengthening of nursing competencies in the community towards the care of vulnerable people.

The second section, entitled Gender-based violence and breastfeeding, is made up of two chapters: chapter six: *prevention, attention and eradication of workplace violence against women*, which reflects on the repercussions on women's health, self-esteem, physical and psychological integrity, freedom and safety, which hinders professional development and equal opportunities at work. In chapter seven: *Breastfeeding rooms, installation and operation,* which visualises breastfeeding at work as a support to increase efficiency and productivity, reduce women's absenteeism because breastfed babies are less likely to get sick, as well as the difficulties that women face at this stage.

The coordinators of the book invite you to read this work, convinced that the chapters will provide elements for consultation as well as a contribution to the professional performance of the readers for the benefit of occupational health.

We would like to express our gratitude to the contributors who reviewed the texts of this work and whose comments, corrections and suggestions helped to ensure the accuracy of the information.

Table of Contents

I. NURSING AND OCCUPATIONAL HEALTH

Chapter 1

Occupational health nursing background

Let the person in charge always keep this question in mind: How can I make the right things always get done? Instead of asking how to do the right thing on their own.

Florence Nightingale

Introduction

The field of occupational health or occupational health is extremely complex and demands the attention of multiple disciplines that, together, achieve the fulfilment of its mission. Nursing fulfils the noble and incredible function, both in this area as in others, the fundamental perspective of health promotion and prevention before the work focused on the curative, therefore, its contribution is highly transcendental. This paper describes the history of nursing in the field of occupational health, its approach and importance, as well as the role of nursing in occupational health and the changes, advances and role of the profession in the field of occupational health, the occupational hazards that staff face and the prevention strategies that the profession has put in place for the health of workers.

According to the World Health Organisation (WHO), occupational health is concerned with the search for maximum well-being at work, both in the practice of work activities and in the consequences that these may have on the health of workers, covering all possible risk levels: physical, mental and social. It also aims to prevent harm to workers caused by the working conditions themselves, insuring and protecting them within their working environment against those risks mentioned that may be harmful to their health. [1]

Occupational health should be primarily an activity focused on the prevention, assessment and control of risks, as well as effective health promotion strategies for the working population. Thus, there is a wide range of skills needed to identify, assess and create strategies for risk control in the workplace, including all categories of risks, as well as health promotion, which is a huge challenge. It is important to note that this is not the work of a single professional group, but a cooperation between different professionals to realise the necessary skills and achieve the goal.

As different bibliographies mention, occupational health is not only about identifying and treating individuals who are already ill, but also about following a series of strategies to prevent illnesses or accidents occurring at work, so that occupational risks are minimised as much as possible. As mentioned above, the team is a multidisciplinary team, as it is a job that requires specific skills at certain times when an occupational situation occurs. Doctors, nurses, occupational hygienists are mostly in charge of health risk minimisation, health promotion and treating or curing the disease when it occurs, while managers, lawyers and labour institutions are in charge of creating strategies for safety improvement, providing adequate protective equipment in the work area, implementing the laws and regulations governing work, respecting the agreements with workers and insuring them, in order to maintain the well-being of the workers. [2]

The professionals who form part of a multidisciplinary occupational health team may be: industrial hygienists, physicians, psychologists, physiotherapists, ergonomists, safety engineers, consultants, work organisation specialists, health economists, academic researchers, and not least, occupational health nurses, all of whom will be discussed in this chapter.

Occupational health nursing background

Nursing is as old as civilisation itself; whenever and wherever people have been sick, wounded or injured and in need of care, there is always a nurse there; during the Middle Ages, this profession was mainly practised by religious orders, spanning from the 16th to the 18th century. [3]

It is worth mentioning that the practice of nursing in Mexico has its antecedents in the well-known Aztec culture, in which the so-called

"Tlamatquiizitl" dedicated her actions to the collective care of health and the environment, enjoying great respect and prestige among the members of the population, Today, she is a character that not only represents the historical background, but also an important figure that can be taken as an example in order to strengthen the leadership of specialists in the field of nursing in their community participation and the valuable work in the maintenance, restoration and improvement of human health. [4]

During colonial times, the various religious orders provided care for the sick. Some of the tasks nurses performed were cures in hospitals and prisons, and they earned 50 pesos a year. They did not need a licence to provide this care. At the end of the 19th century, nurses had a salary of 8 pesos and 25 cents per month and worked long hours: during the day, from 7 am to 8 pm, while at night, from 8 pm to 7 am. On 9 February 1907, the School of Nursing was inaugurated. [5]

In the modern history of the country, nursing played an important role not only in the care of sick and injured people, but also as a disseminator of knowledge to prevent illnesses and protect the health of citizens. The Escuela de Salubridad de México, founded in 1922 and the origin of today's Escuela de Salud Pública de México (ESPM) of the Instituto Nacional de Salud Pública, gave way to professionalisation from a public health perspective with the first "visiting nurse" course in 1925 with 31 students.

The advancement of the nursing profession in occupational health was a gradual step, since it began at the end of the 19th century with the emergence of an industrial nurse: Philipa Flowerday for the firm of J&J Colman in 1878 in England; in this act, the nurse assisted the doctor, visited sick workers and family to their homes. This was the first record of a nurse in occupational health. In 1988, there are records that mention that groups of mining companies hired a nurse, Bety Moulder, to care for sick miners and their families. Later, in 1895, the Vermont-Marble Company hired for the first time an occupational health nurse, Ada Mayo Stewart, accompanied by her sister (who cared for employees in the company's neighbouring branches), becoming the second nurse to be recruited in this field. When the success of nursing services for the health of its employees and work performance was realised, the same company, in 1896, opened a hospital for the benefit of its employees and their families. This led to an increase in the number of industrial nurses in the country. [3]

Between 1910 and 1920, workers' compensation laws and a focus on the prevention of infectious diseases led to the rise of occupational nursing practice. These changes led to the emergence of several occupational nursing organisations. As the years progressed, these organisations were strengthened and their purposes established, which were to improve the practice and education of industrial nurses, to increase inter- and multi-disciplinary collaborative efforts, and to represent the interests of industrial nurses. By 1977, the term "Industrial Nurse" was replaced by "Occupational Health Nurse" improving the scope of practice of nurses in the workplace. [4]

During 1988, the Occupational Safety and Health Association (OSHA) of the United States hired a nurse to provide technical assistance in the development of various statutes and regulations that would regulate occupational health. The above, influenced in such a way, that there was a greater recognition of the contribution of nursing in health in general and specifically in the labour area, this, generated the establishment of the Office of Nursing in Occupational Health in OSHA during 1993, giving a role of higher level and recognition to nursing work, demonstrating the great capacity and importance of this profession in the health of workers, improvement, changes and advances that the contribution had in this area, was a plus for nursing in general. [4]

The main basis for these strategies has been community health and public health, based on the community health model, providing family members with health and community services, as well as industrial health services focused on the prevention and treatment of work-related accidents and diseases.

At present, nursing professionals who started out in the area of occupational health have marked a great path, acquiring greater strength and experience for the changes that have been taking place over the years and continue to advance in this important area of health. It is worth mentioning that this progress is also thanks to events such as the industrial revolution in the 20th century, which allowed nursing practice to broaden its dimensions and from there, new occupational risks began to be recognised.

Introduction to occupational health nursing

Throughout the history of nursing, a great progress has been visualised with respect to the domestic and vocational stages. As we know, from the Middle Ages to the Renaissance, the dark ages of nursing emerged, which were characterised by a deficiency in public health as a result of constant wars, numerous pandemics and therefore high mortality. In these times, women were excluded from social life and relegated to the home, so that delinquents, reas, uneducated people and sex workers were assigned to provide care in this deplorable situation. Until 1907, when the first school for nurses was inaugurated in the General Hospital of Mexico, where the technical and professional stage began, it was here that nursing became known as a scientific discipline. The emergence of nursing in the field of occupational health was gradual and was the result of a process that began at the end of the 19th century. [6]

Specifically, nursing as a profession aims to care for each individual, society, as well as their relationship with their environment. Throughout its history it has had a clear focus on care, self-care and wellbeing which is closely committed to promoting health and, if health has been affected, contributing to its restoration, preventing illness and alleviating suffering so that life regains and maintains an essential value based on humanity and the quality with which care and service delivery are carried out.

In this respect, there are records in different countries which show the recruitment of nursing professionals in different countries in areas of work such as industry, where their main focus is to look after the health of workers.

As far as nursing is concerned, its main area of development and employment is the clinical or care field, in which it seeks to provide quality care in a comprehensive manner in an environment of understanding, comprehension, empathy and reliability with the patient, however, it is necessary to emphasise that the nursing profession is developed in various fields of action, including public health and occupational health. In this respect, the theorists who established the bases for improving the care of nursing professionals, such as Nola J. Pender who developed the health promotion model, Madeleine Leininger who developed and implemented the transcultural theory and Jean Watson who developed the theory of humanism, stand out. All of which can be applicable to occupational health. On the other hand, it is important to talk about Dorothea Orem who, with her self-care deficit theory, also contributed to the foundations of the profession.

As a nursing professional it is important to promote health, to promote healthy habits and a healthy lifestyle and to be aware of risk factors. It is important to pay attention to the work environment without forgetting the training and protocols to follow in any circumstance of risk in order to achieve an assertive communication with workers for the welfare and promotion of self-care.

Current role of nursing in occupational health

The Organisation for Economic Co-operation and Development (OECD) mentions that in Mexico and the world, a large number of health care professionals are required in the workplace. In most nations, there are 6 to 7 nurses per thousand inhabitants, while in Mexico, the proportion is 2.5 per thousand. This number is insufficient for the attention of the citizens. [7]

Unfortunately, in Mexico today, there is little or almost no data on the role of nursing in occupational health, due to the minimal requirement of this profession in workplaces and its diminishing importance.

However, due to the COVID-19 pandemic, nursing was highlighted as a profession, highlighting its importance in preventing, maintaining and restoring the health of individuals, which in a way, could mean a higher level of importance to the nursing profession and its role in community health, opening possible gaps for occupational health. [8]

The functions and areas of action of occupational nursing are varied and broad, seeking to provide holistic and comprehensive care. [9] According to the American Association of Occupational Health Nurses (AAOHN), occupational nursing has a consensus of the different areas of intervention:

Health protection, prevention and promotion: is the main component of occupational health nursing practice which includes activities focused on health promotion and prevention, as well as protection of groups of workers, carrying out primary, secondary and tertiary prevention strategies. They are also responsible for the development of educational programmes to increase employees' knowledge and awareness of exposure to certain occupational hazards, the creation of programmes to promote positive lifestyles (exercise, nutrition, good practices, alcohol and tobacco cessation, etc.), as well as other strategies to promote health-enhancing behaviours and attitudes, and screening for cardiovascular risk or diabetes in order to detect early health problems in employees. The occupational health nurse may also carry out activities focused on legal provisions such as the control of physical, chemical and/or biological hazards in the workplace. In addition, as part of tertiary prevention, she is responsible for the rehabilitation and reintegration of the worker back into the workplace. To this end, it creates an intervention plan that must incorporate physical and psychological care for the affected worker, creating an individual plan for adaptation to their work and activities by restructuring them and retraining the worker, while at the same time motivating the participation of the worker and the employers.

Assessment and diagnosis of workers' health: the occupational health nurse carries out a variety of examinations, monitoring, assessments and other health surveillance activities in which her knowledge is helpful. Here, the nurse must be aware of medical histories and scheduled examinations of each worker, in order to determine the possible adverse effects that the working conditions have brought to health and recommend measures for the correction of these and early identification of chronic diseases. Periodic assessment will allow you to monitor workers who may be exposed to an occupational hazard and maintain their vigilance.

 Surveillance of working conditions and risk detection: staff are involved in monitoring the working environment and developing surveillance programmes in order to identify potential risks to the health of employees. This is done through constant tours of the workplace, familiarising themselves with the activities and therefore with the protective equipment and practices that workers need to maintain their safety. When staff identify a risk, they should measure the levels of exposure, the health impact and the relationship of the risk to the worker, in conjunction with other health professionals.

Primary health care: care is provided for work-related illnesses or injuries already present in the worker, including treatment, follow-up and referral to other areas if required.

Consultancy and advice: this is given to both workers and employers, in order to clarify doubts regarding their well-being and to provide information that helps in decision-making on the issue of well-being and health (for workers); for employers, it consists of advising on the implementation of health services in the company or on problems that require immediate attention in the workplace and for which an expert advisor is likely to be needed.

Management and administrative control: These responsibilities include planning the achievement of departmental goals and objectives, managing the budget, developing policies, practising staff organisation activities, and evaluating occupational health services, as well as creating workplace standards with the help of workers and other professionals.

Research: Nursing plays an important role in research related to workers' health, since knowledge about the health effects of toxins, the identification of the main causes of accidents and illnesses, as well as the factors that produce stress in the worker, are clear examples of occupational health research that have become priority areas.

Ethical-legal framework: the occupational health nursing professional must be aware of the rules, laws and regulations that govern the company where he/she works, as well as those in force in the field of occupational health and safety, in order to enforce them in the workplace and to rely on them when necessary.

Community collaboration: This collaboration enables staff to develop a network of resources to ensure that the services provided by the company and employees are efficient. This can be done with a more community perspective through an awareness of the work environment, which is healthy and also involves health activities aimed at workers' families and the community at large.

After many decades, on 31 January 2018, the University Council of the National Autonomous University of Mexico approved the curriculum for the specialisation in Nursing in Occupational Health, which has the general objective of training nursing professionals specialised in occupational health, who work on the basis of gender needs, ethical principles, scientific knowledge, taking into account national and international standards with skills, abilities and critical and innovative attitudes, in order to provide solutions to the health and safety problems of workers.(10)

Today there are many challenges for occupational health nurses, among which are the shortage of supplies, the lack of knowledge of protocols, official standards and laws that protect and provide security to both the worker and themselves. On the other hand, long working hours, salaries that do not correspond to the work activities and little time for self-improvement are challenges that concern the nursing professional who is dedicated to the occupational area. (11)

Conclusions

With the constant changes and globalisation due to technological development, more adverse working conditions and flexibilities at work, occupational health has become a social need with high demand and higher priority, recognising that its mission, objectives and purposes can only be fulfilled effectively with an inter- and multidisciplinary approach, since, as we saw earlier, it is a very important area that requires the cooperation of different professional areas to achieve its purpose.

Nursing as a profession provides a great and significant contribution to the prevailing challenges of occupational health. Based on theoretical, methodological and philosophical principles, nursing interventions in occupational health have a comprehensive, modern and wide-ranging paradigm for occupational health and safety. The basis of this paradigm emphasises the promotion of health and the prevention of accidents and illnesses in workers, rather than merely focusing on illness. In addition, another aspect that characterises the role of nurses is that they are, in most cases, the first contact with workers on health issues, so they are in a favourable position to attend to the health problems of the aforementioned workers with quality and efficiency.

The interventions and roles of nursing show how important the participation of professionals in this area is, reflected in the establishment of a myriad of organisations, institutions or bodies of nursing practice in occupational health. Thus, the practice of nursing in the area of occupational health, effectively applying primary, secondary and tertiary prevention, allows for the development of the well-being, productivity and quality of life of workers to the benefit of workers, employers and society in general. As discussed in this chapter, nursing has many areas in which to develop in occupational health; it carries out activities that are specific to the profession and others that are not, but those who specialise in this area will acquire knowledge that will support them in the development of occupational nursing competencies and profiles. However, we also came to the conclusion that, despite the importance of occupational nursing, in Mexico there is very little or almost no information on the role of these professionals, due to the fact that it is one of the countries that does not have specialisations of this rank and that there is not much talk about occupational health, it is not given due importance and the recruitment of nursing staff in work centres and companies is only for the purpose of complying with the laws in force, without the staff being trained in this area and expecting them to acquire knowledge by the empirical method.

References

1. Benavides FG, Delclós J, Serra C. Welfare state and public health: the role of occupational health. Gac Sanit [Internet]. 2018;32(4):377-80. Available at: http://dx.doi.org/10.1016/j.gaceta.2017.07.007

2. Moreno Pimentel AG. History of Occupational Nursing in the 19th and mid-20th centuries. Revista Enfermería del Trabajo [Internet]. 2014 [cited 2022 June 17];4(1):14-9. Available from: https://dialnet.unirioja.es/servlet/articulo?codigo=4727948

3. Enfermeriacelayane P. Didactic unit 1A: Generalities [Internet]. Bachelor's degree in Nursing and Midwifery. University System of Educational Multimodality - University of Guanajuato; 2018 [cited 2022 Jun 16]. Available from: https://blogs.ugto.mx/enfermeriaenlinea/unidad-didactica-1-generalidades/

4. Santos A, Arévalo G, García B. Origins of Nursing at Work. Nursing at work. [Internet]. 2014. [Cited June 16, 2022]; IIII: 5-13. Available

from:

http://scholar.google.es/scholar_url?hl=es&q=http://dialnet.unirioja.es/descarga/articulo/4727922.pdf&sa=X&scisig=AAGBfm0IjtgqSbRpHVkD1ICkaaO8ADgyfQ&oi=scholaralrt

5. National Institute of Public Health. Nursing in Mexico, a profession with history. [Internet]. 2020. [Cited September 07, 2022];Available from: https://insp.mx/avisos/4866-dia-enfermeria-historia.html

6. Lourdes Melara Martínez LLMS de ZLM. occupational risks of nursing staff in the infectious disease service of the national children's hospital. [salvador]: university of el salvador faculty of medicine master's degree in hospital management; 2018).

7. Sanabria KVD, editor. The role of the nursing professional in occupational safety and health, innovating care. 2019. [cited 2022 June 17, 2022]. Available from: https://docs.bvsalud.org/biblioref/2021/02/1148066/237.pdf)

8. Figueroa Uribe Augusto Flavio, Hernández Ramírez Julia. Seguridad hospitalaria, una visión de seguridad multidimensional. Rev. Fac. Med. Hum. [Internet]. 2021 Jan [cited 2022 Jun 17] ; 21(1): 169-178. Available from: http://www.scielo.org.pe/scielo.php?script=sci_arttext&pid=S2308-05312021000100169&lng=es. http://dx.doi.org/10.25176/rfmh.v21i1.3490.)

9. Elsevier. Occupational Nursing, a speciality with many possibilities [Internet]. Elsevier Connect. [cited 2022 Jun 29, 2022]. Available from: https://www.elsevier.com/es-es/connect/enfermeria/enfermeria-del-trabajo,-una-especialidad-con-muchas-posibilidades

10. De Estudios F, Iztacala S, Especialista En Enfermería• ., Laboral S. UNIVERSIDAD NACIONAL AUTÓNOMA DE MÉXICO [Internet]. Unam.mx. [cited 29 June 2022]. Available from: https://www.posgrado.unam.mx/oferta/planes/e2/PP_Esp_Enfer_Salud_Laboral-Tomo_I.pdf

11. Aguirre Raya Dalila Aida. Challenges of nursing in the modern world. Rev haban cienc méd [Internet]. 2020 Jun [cited 2022 Jun

29] ; 19(3): e3229. Available from: http://scielo.sld.cu/scielo.php?script=sci_arttext&pid=S1729-519X2020000300001&lng=es. Epub 10-Jul-2020.

Chapter 2

Nursing organisations promoting occupational health.

Nurses have that unique and insatiable way of caring for others, which is both a great strength and a weakness.

Dr. Jean Watson

Introduction

Nursing is a profession that has evolved over time, adapting to the social changes that are taking place, not only in the acquisition of theory and fundamentals that enhance it, but also in the health of workers and that they have the necessary means to be able to work effectively.

Let us recall that occupational health is defined as a multidisciplinary action that aims to holistically cover the integrity of workers, i.e. it promotes and maintains a state of physical, mental and social well-being of workers.

Occupational health is a concept that has also been gaining importance in recent times; this is reflected in the creation of both national and international organisations that focus on improving the labour sector, as well as caring for the well-being of workers.

Even in occupational health, the discipline of nursing is reflected in the publication of Order SAS/1348/2009, which was the first to approve a training programme for occupational nursing. This defined a new action protocol based on promoting competences acquired in the fields of prevention, care, legal and expert, management, teaching and research. In this specific development of its professional competences, the article explores the added value for organisations of developing interventions with a preventive approach in the workplace by this nursing speciality, the impact of which has been noted by various institutions.

The following chapter will deal with the different nursing organisations that promote occupational health, but the research will not only focus on them, but will also investigate both national and international organisations, with the aim of making a list of these organisations and the role they play in occupational health.

International organisations

International Labour Organisation (ILO)

One of the major labour organisations, a tripartite agency of the UN, the ILO is made up of government, employers and workers. It is made up of 187 members whose aim is to formulate policies and develop programmes promoting labour rights, foster decent work opportunities, improve social protection and strengthen dialogue in addressing labour-related issues.[1]

The way in which this body takes decisions is peculiar in that it has a tripartite structure, in which the workers and employers have equal voting rights with the state during deliberations to ensure that the views of the social partners are accurately reflected in the ILO's standards, policies and programmes.

The International Labour Organisation in its 2019 document "The rules of the game" talks about occupational safety and health; it establishes the principle that workers must be protected against illnesses in general or occupational diseases and accidents resulting from their work, but it is known that this is not fully complied with, as it is far from reality. This is why the ILO imposes fundamental principles on occupational safety and health, for example in 2006, when the "Convention on the Promotional Framework for Occupational Safety and Health" was drawn up with the aim of providing a coherent and systematic treatment of occupational safety and health issues and to promote the recognition of related conventions. However, it does not only focus on recognition, but also covers the working environment, where the working environment must comply with hygiene standards, as well as the respect of safety in different work sectors such as mines, construction, agriculture, etc. Finally, recommendations for risk control in radiation, occupational cancer, working environment, asbestos and chemicals. [1]

Moreover, in its report on the application of international standards 2022, which covers the overview of the ILO's supervisory mechanisms, the functions of international labour standards and the repercussions of the HIV/AIDS pandemic left behind are addressed. It also discusses the observations on concepts such as job security, wages, forced labour, child labour, occupational safety and health, among others. [2]

American Association of Occupational Health Nurses (AAONH)

It is the professional association of licensed nurses engaged in the practice of occupational and environmental health nursing. The primary roles and responsibilities of AAOHN are[3] :

1. Define scope of practice and set standards for occupational and environmental health nurses.
2. Develop standards of professional conduct for occupational and environmental nursing as outlined in the AAOHN Code of Ethics.
3. Promote the health and safety of working and working communities.
4. Promote and provide continuing learning opportunities for nurses and occupational and environmental health professionals offered through the AAOHN Academy.
5. Advance the profession by encouraging and facilitating research. Advocate for occupational and environmental health nursing in business, hospitals, government and other professional areas.
6. Responding to issues critical to occupational and environmental nursing practice

Occupational Safety and Health Association (OSHA)

This association was created by the US Congress to ensure that all employees work in safe and healthy conditions through the establishment and enforcement of standards and training, outreach programmes and activities, education and compliance assistance. It covers the whole of the United States and, like the STPS in Mexico, it promotes the regulations and also monitors that they are respected in order to preserve the integrity and freedom of the employee[3] .

The programmes it manages and which are available to everyone are the following:

- Filing a complaint
  Either online or by phone, mail, email or fax sent to the nearest OSHA office and workers can request an inspection. If working conditions at a site are not safe and healthful.

- Whistleblower protection programme
  In order for workers to be free to participate in safety and health activities, the law prohibits a person from dismissing or retaliating against a worker for claiming rights protected by the law.

- In case of a dangerous work situation

If a worker believes that working conditions are unsafe and unhealthy, OSHA recommends that he or she tell the employer, if possible. A worker may file a complaint with OSHA about an unsafe working condition at any time. However, he or she should not leave the workplace simply because a complaint has been filed. Obviously, if the situation presents a risk of death or serious physical harm, if there is no time for OSHA to make an inspection, and if, where possible, the worker has notified the employer of the situation, the worker may have a statutory right to refuse to work in a situation in which he or she could be exposed to the hazard.

American Board of Occupational Health Nurses (ABOHN)

The American Board of Occupational Health Nurses (ABOHN) is an independent nursing specialty certification board and was founded in 1972 as an independent non-profit organisation to establish professional standards and conduct occupational health nursing specialty certification. ABOHN is the only certifying body for occupational health nurses in the United States and awards three credentials[4] :

1. Certified Occupational Health Nurse (COHN)
2. Certified Occupational Health Nurse Specialist (COHN-S)
3. Case management (CM)

The possibility of certification of occupational health nurses had been investigated for several years. In 1969, the American Association of Industrial Nurses formed a committee called the Interorganisational Committee for the Certification of Occupational Health Nurses to investigate and recommend a course of action regarding certification. Upon hearing the recommendation of the Interorganisational Committee, the American Board of Occupational Health Nurses (ABOHN) was established on May 21, 1971. The joint committee was composed of representatives from the American Association of Industrial Nurses (AAIN), the American Academy of Occupational Medicine (AAOM), the Industrial Medical Association (IMA), the American Industrial Hygiene Association (AIHA) and the American Association of Industrial Nurses Advisory Council. [4]

American Association of Occupational Health Nurses (AAOHN)

The rise of occupational health nursing practice between 1910 and 1920 was accelerated by the advent of workers' compensation laws and the emphasis on prevention of infectious diseases. Several prominent organisations related to occupational health nursing began to be founded, among them the Industrial Nursing Section of the American Nurses Association (ANA). This section eventually evolved into an independent association: the American Association of Industrial Nurses (AAIN). In 1942, the purposes of the AAIN were formally delineated to include the improvement of industrial nursing education and practice, the enhancement of collaborative, interdisciplinary efforts, and to truly represent the interests of industrial nurses.[5]

In 1977 the AAIN changed its name to the American Association of Occupational Health Nurses (AAOHN). The term "Occupational Health Nurse" replaces the term "Industrial Nurse" to better reflect the broad scope of practice of nurses in this field. [5]

The association also defines occupational health as "the specialty that provides and delivers health care services to workers". The practice focuses on the protection, promotion and restoration of workers' health within the context of a safe and healthy work environment. Occupational health nursing practice is independent and autonomous in the provision of occupational health services. Its practice is research-based with an emphasis on health optimisation, disease and injury prevention and health risk reduction.

National Agencies

Ministry of Labour and Social Security (STPS)

It is an agency of the Federal Government that focuses on verifying compliance with the labour rights of workers and their families, in order to guarantee their health integrity. It also builds democratic relations between employers and workers through the use of effective communication.[6]

This national department develops different programmes for the general public where you can see transparency, solve worker and employer problems, among others. However, the STPS offers a General Organisation Manual of the Ministry of Labour and Social Welfare, whose objective is to inform about the mission, vision and objectives of this agency, as well as its historical background; the legal framework on which its actions are based; the basic organisational structure and the powers of its administrative units and decentralised administrative bodies. [6]

Its priority objectives are as follows:

1. Achieving the inclusion of young people through on-the-job training.

2. Promote social dialogue, trade union democracy and genuine collective bargaining in line with the new labour model.
3. Restore the purchasing power of minimum wages and incomes to improve the quality of life of workers.
4. Dignify work and stimulate productivity by monitoring compliance with labour regulations.
5. To achieve the insertion into formal employment of unemployed people, workers in critical conditions of occupation and inactive people who are available for work, with preferential attention to those who face barriers to access formal employment. [7]

It is also important to mention that the STPS stipulates all regulations related to safety at work. Specifically, it issues Mexican Official Standards (NOM), which can be distinguished by having the acronym of the Ministry of Labour in its name. For example, NOM-002-STPS-2001. Among the most important norms are:

NOM-002-STPS-1993: This specifies the appropriate conditions for handling and preventing fires.
NOM-015-STPS-1994: Discusses the Personal Protective Equipment (PPE) that employees need while in the workplace.
NOM-027-STPS-1994: This standard provides guidelines on how to develop health and safety signs and notices.

Standing Committee on Nursing (SCC)

The Permanent Nursing Commission is an advisory body of the Ministry of Health, whose objective is to analyse and conduct the activities undertaken in the field of nursing, in order to help improve the efficiency and quality of health care services, their adequate development and the training and improvement of nursing personnel. [8]

Likewise, it will be the body that will have a positive impact on the level of health of the population, by favouring excellence in the provision of nursing services based on the principles of equality, coverage, accessibility and sustainability in the quality and training of its professionals.

The basic process is summarised in a modular care that ensures a specialised and personalised service by competent medical and legal staff; it applies standardised and certified processes under the ISO 9001:2000 standard, which the institution fully endorses every six months before a certifying agency, in accordance with the institutional regulations and procedures, within the framework of civil law and the corresponding codes. Both parties, defendant and plaintiff, must voluntarily undertake the institutional procedure, which begins with the filing of the medical complaint. This submission involves the institutional receipt of a complaint for a medical act performed, in which there is a suspicion of possible malpractice in the surgical or medical provision, where there must be some unexpected result or some objective negative consequence, whether financial or physical; and that both parties, once the procedure is understood, empowers the institution to act, according to the situation at the basis of the controversy. [8]

CONAMED

The National Medical Arbitration Commission is an organ of the Ministry of Health, established by presidential decree, published in the Official Journal of the Federation on 3 June 1996, to contribute to the protection of the right to health protection and to improve the quality of medical services. [9]

CONAMED is a specialised body with technical autonomy and powers to receive accusations, investigate alleged irregularities in the provision of medical services and issue its opinions or agreements, which allow for the resolution of conflicts acting with confidentiality, impartiality and respect, through alternative procedures for the resolution of conflicts such as: guidance, immediate management, conciliation and arbitration.

It is important to note which issues CONAMED deals with, among these are:

Acts or omissions arising from the provision of health services, as well as alleged acts of possible malpractice with consequences for the health of the user, which strictly speaking means that it only deals with problems related to such services or the refusal to provide them.

Among the issues it does not address are[10] :

1. Acts or omissions constituting an offence(s)

2. Cases already pending before other civil courts.

3. Labour disputes or competences of the labour authorities in the field of social security.

4. Cases whose purpose is to obtain pre-constituted evidence for the initiation of legal proceedings.

5. When the sole purpose is to sanction the medical service provider.

Conclusions

With globalisation and the constant alterations in production processes characterised by technological growth, labour flexibilisation and more adverse working conditions, occupational health has become a social necessity of vital importance, recognising that its mission and objectives can only be fulfilled with a multi- and interdisciplinary approach.

The interventions and roles of the nurse in occupational health show the important participation of the discipline in this field, a fact that is also reflected in the institution and establishment of a large number of associations or organisations of nurses applied to occupational health, especially in developed countries, where the outstanding contribution of the profession has been important and its growth is evident. In Europe and the United States, nurses are the occupational group with the largest number of people providing occupational health services in companies, and in some countries, their practice is even required by law.

In Mexico, occupational health has been a field almost belonging to the medical profession, with little participation of nurses' associations in occupational health, and there are few educational programmes focused on this speciality, which implies an emerging need to be covered in the coming years, which will undoubtedly be driven by the social demands that are to come.

In addition to this, thanks to the research carried out, we were able to realise how little information and formality there is regarding nursing organisations that promote occupational health, especially in our country, since in addition to the fact that very few institutions exist, they are described in a very general and vague way, which detracts a lot from the importance of this type of issue.

References

1. About the ILO. [cited 2022 Jun 16]; Available from: https://www.ilo.org/global/about-the-ilo/lang--es/index.htm

2. International Labour Organization. Application of international labour standards, 2022 [internet]. Geneva 2022 [accessed 15 June 2022]. Available at: https://www.ilo.org/wcmsp5/groups/public/---ed_norm/---relconf/documents/meetingdocument/wcms_836655.pdf

3. American Association of Occupational Health Nurses. About AAOHN [internet]. EU; 2020 [accessed June 15, 2022]. Available from:http://aaohn.org/page/about-aaohn

4. History [Internet]. Abohn.org. 2022 [cited 2022 Jun 16]. Available from: https://www.abohn.org/about-abohn/history

5. Occupational Safety and Health Association. All About OSHA [internet]. EU; 2020 [accessed 15 June 2022]. Available from: https://www.osha.gov/sites/default/files/publications/osha3173.pdf

6. Secretaría del Trabajo y Previsión Social, What are we doing [internet]. Mexico; 2020 [accessed 15 June 2022]. Available from: https://www.gob.mx/stps/que-hacemos; 2021

7. Esoarza J.A. What are the functions of the Ministry of Labour and Social Welfare? [internet]. Mexico. [accessed 5 September 2022]. Available at: https://www.sesamehr.mx/blog/cuales-son-las-funciones-de-la-secretaria-del-trabajo-y-prevision-social/

8. Standing Commission on Nursing CPE [Internet]. 2021 [cited 2022 June 16]. Available from: http://www.cpe.salud.gob.mx/

9. National Medical Arbitration Commission [Internet]. 2022 [cited 2022 June 16]. Available from: https://www.sesamehr.mx/blog/cuales-son-las-funciones-de-la-secretaria-del-trabajo-y-prevision-social/http://www.conamed.gob.mx/gobmx/prevencion/intro.php

10. National Medical Arbitration Commission. Information on CONAMED for health professionals. [Internet]. 2022 [cited 2022 Sep 08]. Available from: http://www.conamed.gob.mx/prof_salud/pdf/funciones.pdf

11. International Labour Organisation. Rules of the game [internet]. Geneva 2019 [accessed 15 June 2022]. Available from:https://www.ilo.org/wcmsp5/groups/public/---ed_norm/---normes/documents/publication/wcms_672554.pdf

12. Ministry of Labour and Social Welfare. Manual de Organización General de la Secretaría del Trabajo y Previsión Social. [internet]. Mexico; 2021 [accessed 15 June 2022]. Available at: https://dof.gob.mx/2021/STPS/MOG_STPS_070421.pdf

13. Juárez A, Hernández E. Nursing interventions in occupational health [Internet]. 2022 [cited 2022 June 16, 2022]. Available from: https://www.medigraphic.com/pdfs/enfermeriaimss/eim-2010/eim101e.pdf

Chapter 3

Nursing intervention in occupational health

To be in charge is not only to execute the appropriate measures but also to check that others do so as well, to see that no one deliberately or unintentionally does anything that could undermine those measures.

Florence Nightingale.

Introduction

According to the International Labour Organisation (ILO), it is estimated that 1,000 people die every day in the world due to occupational accidents and another 6,500 due to occupational diseases. The impact is quantified in terms of compensation, lost working days, material damage, administrative sanctions, liability claims, interruptions in the production process, healthcare costs, loss of qualified personnel and professional retraining, among others. [1]

One of the functions of the nursing staff in charge of occupational health is to assess the main risks and harm to which workers are exposed and from there to carry out proactive strategies that help to prevent and control these harms. For this reason, they must carry out activities specifically aimed at promoting the health of this working population, from the most basic aspects such as healthy lifestyle habits, to carrying out different training according to their roles, as well as instilling the reporting of unexpected events and acting in accordance with appropriate behaviours. [2]

In order to carry out this type of intervention, it is necessary for the nursing staff in charge to find out about the activities carried out in the work area (companies, factories, etc.) and to be observant so that they are aware of the main consequences and risks that the worker may suffer during their working day, in order to provide the best possible safety and maximum well-being in their work area.

In this area of health, the role of the nursing staff is based on Primary Health Care through activities aimed at health promotion, such as: Providing information to workers and mainly to the heads of the work areas about the different activities and measures to be considered in the work area in order to prevent and control accidents.

It is also important to mention that the responsibility for occupational health does not only fall on those professionals in nursing, as the work area lends itself to be multidisciplinary and therefore must work together with other professionals such as engineers with different approaches, doctors and psychologists, who work permanently in prevention, promotion and in the curative part, primarily for the needs of these subjects in order to maintain greater productivity, and thus be effective in their work by preserving their health. By this we can refer to the fact that workers can suffer not only physical but also psychological damage, i.e. damage to their mental health, either due to work-related stress, long working hours or extensive work demands.

In other words, nursing plays a very important role in the area of occupational health, because in order to participate and perform in the best possible way, it is necessary to take into account not only the physical part of the workers but also the mental health and the social area, as this is also affected if one of the aforementioned is deficient. For a person to be in good health, he or she must have a certain level of physical, mental and social well-being in order to be able to function in a way that allows him or her to fulfil all personal and work-related functions, hence the importance of addressing this issue. This chapter deals with the different scenarios in which the discipline of nursing intervenes in relation to occupational health, identifying the role of these professionals and the different activities they carry out.

Scenarios for occupational health nursing intervention

The American Association of Occupational Health Nurses (AAOHN) defines Occupational Health Nursing as "The application of nursing principles to the preservation of the health of workers in all occupations". From this definition, it can be said that occupational nursing is concerned with protecting the working population from health problems, illnesses and injuries arising from their work activities, which are a major concern of international labour organisations. [3]

The main objective of occupational health is to ensure the well-being, health and working conditions of every individual in an organisation. The presence of occupational health in an organisation is of vital importance because in addition to providing for the highest physical, mental and social well-being of employees, it also seeks to establish and sustain a safe and healthy working environment. It is therefore a commitment to create a sufficiently effective occupational health programme that provides safety, security and comprehensive care to employees so that they can perform their jobs and generate more productivity. [4]

Due to the importance of occupational health, the services provided must have as their main objective the prevention of illnesses or accidents that may occur at work. This can be achieved through preventive and health promotion programmes, where the main tool will be the evaluation and observation of the work area.

As is well known, the nursing professional plays an important role in all health services, both curative and preventive; in fact, with training and qualification, he/she can manage health services with minimal medical support. In occupational health this is no different, as nursing is also an emerging area of specialisation.

In accordance with the above, nursing is an essential pillar of the occupational health team as it addresses the state of health of individuals in their relationship with the work environment, with the main objective of achieving the highest degree of physical, mental and social well-being of the working population, taking into account the individual characteristics of the worker, the workplace and the socio-occupational environment in which he/she works. [5]

Because occupational health is not just about identifying and treating individuals who have become ill, but about taking all necessary steps to prevent cases of work-related illness, areas of opportunity have been found and classified in which nurses can intervene.

With reference to the above, the main areas of intervention for nurses in occupational health cover the following[6] :

- Health protection, prevention and promotion
- Assessment and diagnosis of workers' health
- Monitoring of working conditions and risk detection
- Primary health care
- Consultancy and advice
- Management and administrative control of occupational health
- Research
- Ethical and legal framework
- Community collaboration

This section includes some of the activities carried out by the occupational health nurse:

- Opening and management of workers' medical and employment records.
- Development and review of protocols for surveillance and control of worker health.
- Prospective surveillance of the health of workers
- Care for workers in special situations
- Development of immunisation and prophylaxis programme for workers at risk.
- Establishment of criteria for work restrictions for workers due to communicable diseases.

- Register of occupational accidents, occupational diseases and work-related diseases.
- Study of absenteeism due to accidents at work, occupational diseases, work-related diseases and common contingencies.
- Occupational epidemiology: Study of work-related pathologies.
- Work-related health promotion
- Collaboration in carrying out the assessment of working conditions
- Collaboration in the assessment of personal protection equipment
- Health planning.

Health protection, prevention and promotion

Health promotion represents an important role for nurses, which aims to prevent, counteract and mitigate harm in particular. In the case of occupational health, it is aimed especially at those individuals who fulfil the role of worker, creating strategies based on the different levels of prevention; primary, secondary and tertiary. [2]

Thus, the activities carried out by these professionals allow the development and implementation of programmes aimed at education to raise awareness of the different risk exposures in which they are immersed daily in the work environment, whether physical, chemical or biological. Likewise, the creation of workshops on personal care issues covering healthy eating, healthy lifestyles, addiction control and behavioural management, as well as awareness and early detection of cardiovascular problems.

On the other hand, nursing professionals are also in charge of the reintegration into the labour market of those workers who went through certain situations in which their health was affected, incorporating strategies for the physical and mental care of the person.[5]

In addition to general health care, all workers, and particularly those in high-risk occupations, need health services that assess and reduce exposure to occupational hazards, as well as medical surveillance services for the early detection of occupational and work-related diseases and injuries. [6]

Assessment and diagnosis of workers' health

The nurse in charge of occupational health must first identify and determine the general health status of all workers. To do this, it is necessary to carry out certain types of assessments, examinations, monitoring and other health surveillance activities, so their knowledge in the area will be helpful in providing a proper diagnosis and providing the necessary and required care. [7]

Assessments should be carried out on an ongoing basis to monitor existing risks. These assessments are of great help in determining what are the main adverse health effects that have occurred throughout the working day as a result of the conditions in which workers work. The final result of the assessments allows the health personnel to recommend preventive measures for the timely identification of possible diseases and risks to which the workers are exposed.[7]

The assessment is part of a medical surveillance programme that serves to monitor workers who are at risk from exposure to chemical or toxic substances in the work environment. This means that the nursing professional must know and take into account the medical records of the workers, as they contain all the necessary information in case medical attention is required. This information includes identification data, blood type, previously diagnosed illnesses (HT, DM, HIV/AIDS, Hepatitis, etc.), whether the patient is under treatment for certain pathologies, allergies, hereditary and family history, habits, disabilities, immunisations, physical examinations and the evolution of the patient, among other data that are important for the nursing staff when providing care.

Monitoring of working conditions and risk detection

The nursing staff in charge must be familiar with the work environment, which is why it is essential that they are familiar with the different departments, processes and practices that are carried out within them in order to identify risks to the working staff. In such a way, it is necessary to have close monitoring programmes in place, carrying out inspections, tours and identifying imminent risks to the health of the individual in conjunction with the multidisciplinary staff of the company or organisation in question. They will also be responsible for analysing the data in order to implement strategies for the control, prevention and care of workers' health. [5]

Primary health care

It is important that workplaces have a department or space especially for the nursing professional, because regardless of the occupation people are always exposed to different occupational hazards, therefore a dedicated place for health care is always required.

Because the care provided is specifically directed towards injuries acquired during the working day, nurses can also attend to cases not directly related to the work area, e.g. less serious disease processes such as influenza, stomach illnesses and various other symptomatology. [2]

Consultancy and advice

It is important to emphasise that advice and training should not only be given to the staff (employee) but also to the employer (boss), as both have a responsibility to know what action to take in case of adverse events and accidents. [3]

Likewise, in order to provide information to the employee, it must first be designed in a way that can be understood and clarify doubts regarding their well-being. The information provided should be helpful in making decisions for the safety of employees. The nurse should provide assistance and guidance to employees so that they are able to seek timely medical assistance and treat any health problems.

With reference to employers, they are the ones who should be trained and provided with information so that in their work areas they are able to implement health measures and services that are competent when dealing with problems or situations that require immediate medical attention in the workplace, which makes it important to have an expert advisor to provide care. [3]

Management and administrative control of occupational health

Nursing staff assume a great responsibility in the management and administrative control of health services in companies, as they are in charge of the fulfilment of the different goals set from the beginning and of the objectives of the department, as well as of the financial part destined to this area, they carry out activities of organisation and coordination of personnel, as well as the evaluation of occupational health services. [3]

On the other hand, they also play the role of quality improvement, which requires analysis and inspections to identify areas of opportunity in the workspace.

Research

One of the four pillars of nursing is research and in this speciality of occupational health it is also involved, so it is necessary to stress its importance. [2]

Occupational health nurses play the role of investigators, as it is essential that they find out what are the effects caused by exposures to micro-organisms and toxic substances on workers. It is also important to take into account those illnesses caused by working hours, whether due to excessive working hours or accidents, and the repercussions they have on workers and their work activities. [3]

With reference to the above, research is not only to investigate in different platforms and bibliographies to understand and know how to treat them, but also to go deeper, and in this case the occupational health nurse is in charge of carrying out research with the working staff by identifying, collecting data and making detailed records of those abnormal events that are identified, such as continuous illnesses, injuries and other events that affect the development of the individual in the work area. [2]

Ethical and legal framework

The obligations of occupational health professionals include protecting the life and health of workers, respecting human dignity and promoting the highest ethical principles in occupational health policies and programmes. Integrity in professional conduct, impartiality and the protection of confidentiality of workers' health data and privacy are also part of these obligations. [8]

As a primary requirement of companies or factories that provide employment, they have a statutory responsibility to provide a safe and healthy working environment for workers through the implementation of programmes that contribute to achieving the goal of occupational health. [7]

For this reason, the nursing professional must be aware of the laws and regulations that are in force in the country with reference to occupational health and safety. For example, in Mexico, the health personnel in charge of occupational health must know the provisions established in the Political Constitution of the United Mexican States, in the Federal Labour Law, in the Social Security Law, in the Safety, Hygiene and Work Environment Regulations and in other legal documents of the country. All of these provisions are necessary for proper occupational health.

One of the regulations published in the Official Journal of the Federation establishes the provisions on Occupational Safety and Health that must be observed in workplaces, in order to have the conditions to prevent risks and thus guarantee workers the right to carry out their activities in environments that ensure their life and health, based on the provisions of the Federal Labour Law. [9]

Community collaboration

Collaboration between community groups and organisations undoubtedly makes it easier for nurses to create a network of support and resources to deliver their services to both employers and employees efficiently.

These services should not only focus on the physical and personal well-being of the employee, but should also integrate into their care the social side of the worker by taking into account activities related to the health of the families and other people around each of these workers.

The Community Strategy attaches particular importance to encouraging the development and implementation of national health and safety strategies. To a large extent, the success of the Community strategy will depend on a clear commitment by Member States to adopt coherent national strategies setting quantitative targets for reducing accidents at work and occupational diseases. Such strategies should be targeted at the worst performing sectors and enterprises, and focus on the most common risks and the most vulnerable workers. The definition of such strategies should be based on a detailed assessment of the national situation, with the active involvement and consultation of all stakeholders, in particular the social partners.[10]

The promotion of behavioural change has a prominent place: a strategy aimed at promoting a culture of prevention must address all components of society and not be limited to the workplace and the working population. It must contribute to creating a general culture that attaches the utmost importance to health and risk prevention. In this perspective, the integration of health and safety in education and training programmes at all levels of the education cycle and in all areas, including vocational training and universities, is of paramount importance. [10]

Conclusions

As has been shown in this chapter, the nursing professional plays an important role in the area of work, being in charge of identifying and attending to health problems caused at work. On the other hand, they also participate in various areas of the workplace, such as administration, prevention, care, education, research and management, thus covering the needs of these subjects of care, guaranteeing greater productivity and therefore efficiency and effectiveness in maintaining their health.

Occupational health and healthy work environments are considered important among individuals, communities and countries. Simply put, a healthy work environment is essential, not only for the health of workers, but also for achieving a positive contribution to productivity, work motivation, work ethos, satisfaction and overall quality of life.

The care provided by nursing staff covers different contexts, as it is not only oriented towards the individual, but also encompasses collectives, as in this case, the company. They intervene in the fields of health promotion, prevention and control of illnesses in workers at company level, identifying risk factors in order to reduce accidents at work and the appearance of occupational illnesses, promoting healthy habits and specific protective actions in workers through the development of preventive programmes at occupational level led by nursing staff.

In short, every day there are more and more areas in which the nursing professional can develop, as they are not only involved in care, but there are also areas of opportunity in which they can contribute. Their roles and interventions should not be limited, as it has been demonstrated that they have the capacity to adapt to changes, always bearing in mind their main objective, which is to look after the person with a health deviation in any space, in this case, the work area.

References

1. González-Caballero Javier. Occupational nursing with a holistic perspective. Arco Prev Occupational Risks [Internet]. 2021 Jun

[cited 2022 Sep 09]; 24(2): 175-184. Available from: http://scielo.isciii.es/scielo.php?script=sci_arttext&pid=S1578-25492021000200175&lng=es. Epub 11 Oct 2021. https://dx.doi.org/10.12961/aprl.2021.24.02.08.

2. Ramírez, A. V. Occupational health services. An. Fac. Med. [Internet]. 2012 [Cited June 11, 2022]; 73(1), 63-69. Available from: https://doi.org/10.15381/anales.v73i1.814

3. Peruvian Congress of Occupational Health. Training of the Nurse in Occupational Health. New scenarios [Internet]. Miranda; 2020. [cited 12 June 2022]. Available from: https://docplayer.es/15156380-Formacion-de-la-enfermera-en-salud-ocupacional-nuevos-escenarios.html

4. Ascendo. The importance of occupational health in organisations. [Internet]. 2022. [cited 2022 September 08, 2022]. Available from: https://blog.acsendo.com/la-importancia-de-la-salud-ocupacional-en-las-organizaciones.

5. Gómez-Rojas, ML., Laguado-Jaimes, E. Propuesta de intervención de enfermeria de los factores de riesgo que afectan un entorno laboral. Redalyc.org [Internet]. 2013 [Cited June 12, 2022]; 4 (1): 557-563. Available from: https://www.redalyc.org/pdf/3595/359533224018.pdf

6. World Health Organisation. Protecting the health of workers. [Internet]. 2017. [cited 2022 Sep 08]. Available from: https://www.who.int/es/news-room/fact-sheets/detail/protecting-workers'-health.

7. Juárez-García A., Hernández-Mendoza E. Nursing interventions in occupational health. Medigraphic.com [Internet]. 2010 [Cited June 11, 2022]; 18 (1): 23-29. Available from: https://www.medigraphic.com/pdfs/enfermeriaimss/eim-2010/eim101e.pdf

8. International Commission on Occupational Health. Code of ethics for occupational health professionals, December 1991. [Internet]. 2001. Lat. Rev. Occupational health. 1 (2); [cited 2022 Sep 08].

Available from: https://www.medigraphic.com/pdfs/trabajo/lm-2001/lm012b.pdf

9. Official Journal of the Federation. Reglamento Federal de Seguridad y Salud en el Trabajo. [Internet]. 2014. [cited 08 September 2022]. Available from: https://www.dof.gob.mx/nota_detalle.php?codigo=5368114&fecha=13/11/2014#gsc.tab=0

10. Álvarez Hidalgo Francisco Jesús. The community strategy for health and safety at work 2007 - 2012: a step forward in the protection of European workers. Med. segur. trab. [Internet]. 2007 Jun [cited 2022 September 09]; 53(207).Available from:http://scielo.isciii.es/scielo.php?script=sci_arttext&pid=S0465-546X2007000200001&lng=es.

Chapter 4

Occupational health nursing challenges

The nurse's sole function is to assist the individual, healthy or ill, in the performance of those activities that contribute to health or recovery (or a peaceful death), activities that he or she would perform unaided if he or she had the strength, will and knowledge.

Virginia Henderson

Introduction

Work is a basic human right, through which daily life is sustained and, of course, satisfies basic needs, especially those that go beyond the physical, as it is also the means by which individuals face society, their families and even their identities. It is in this context that, since 2004, the International Labour Organisation (ILO) has been calling on most of the world's nations to seek strategies to ensure the well-being of workers and to propose solutions to "specific problems" with the aim of generating decent work, in order to raise labour productivity, growth and well-being at work.[1]

Health personnel are those involved in activities focused on health recovery and are comprised of doctors, nurses, midwives, laboratory personnel, auxiliary personnel and social workers, who provide their services on a daily basis for the functioning of the health system. [2]

Nursing in the 20th century faces great difficulties and challenges that mark the way forward not only from a practical but also from an ethical point of view. Various historical, political, demographic, demographic, cultural, economic and technological developments have influenced nursing practice to the present day.

Some of the relevant events where health personnel were present were the struggles for justice and social awareness during the two world wars where hospital nurses played a vital role in saving millions of lives through their dedication and care. Add to this the racial conflicts, the national liberation movements in Latin America and Africa, the atomic bombings of Hiroshima and Nagasaki that caused massive death tolls and their consequences still linger to this day.[2]

These facts are somehow related to another important event that needs to be pointed out, which is mediated by the coverage, availability and quality of nursing care for the world's population: genetic phenomena large migrations from Central and South America northwards from the continent or other parts of the world in search of higher salary opportunities and better working conditions for medical professionals and technicians.[2]

Another challenge facing health personnel are the changes in health policy, the introduction of innovations in hospitals, in medical technology, the reorientation of diagnosis-oriented medicine towards preventive practices and with it the strengthening of nursing competencies in the community towards the care of vulnerable people.

Due to the nature of the work carried out by health personnel and especially nursing professionals, they are exposed to a series of risks related to the multiple activities they carry out, whether they are dependent, interdependent or independent, as these can affect their health and safety if preventive measures and protocols are not put into practice to reduce the damage, and it is important to mention in this chapter the chemical, physical, biological and psychosocial risks that can affect the health of the aforementioned personnel. [3]

Nursing in occupational health

Industrial nursing, sometimes called occupational nursing or occupational health nursing, is a branch of nursing whose purpose is the preservation of workers' health, prevention and care of occupational accidents, occupational diseases and rehabilitation, through programmes that not only reach workers, but also the population surrounding these work areas.[4]

In this sense, an important aspect to consider is the monitoring of the state of health of workers, the adequate and correct recording, observation and analysis of the health data of each worker, in an essential clinical-work history, make up a large number of activities and work procedures in which the Workplace Nurse Specialists must intervene, act and decide. [5]

Therefore, occupational health is a prevention-oriented activity, focused on risk assessment and control, as well as on the implementation of proactive strategies aimed at health promotion in the working population.[6]

It should be noted that nursing is as old as civilisation itself; at any time and in any place where people needed care because they were sick, injured or wounded, there was always a nurse present. [5] Community health and public health are the pillars on which this field is based. Early nurses in industry based their practice on community health models, providing family and community health services, as well as industrial health services focused on the prevention and treatment of work-related illnesses and accidents.

That is, occupational nursing practice derives from a synthesis of knowledge drawn primarily from medicine, public health, social sciences, management theories and labour law.

Within the framework of the above considerations, the American Association of Occupational Health Nurses (AAOHN) defines the practice of the occupational health nurse as: "the specialty that provides and delivers health care services to workers. Its practice focuses on the promotion, protection, and restoration of workers' health within the context of a safe and healthful work environment.[6]

In Mexico, occupational health has been an almost exclusive field of the medical profession with little participation of occupational health nursing associations and it should be noted that there are even few educational programmes focused on this speciality, which implies an emerging need that will have to be covered in the coming years. In this sense, the future is full of challenges for the occupational health nurse.

Environmental risks in the area of health

Occupational risk is a series of factors that easily lead to accidents, affecting the physical and mental health of employees. Different groups of professionals face risks at work depending on the area in which they carry out their daily activities. Many of these vary depending on the different environments, with some being more common in other occupations, such as biological-infectious accidents being more specific or frequent in health care workers due to the nature of their work areas. Risks can be classified as follows[3] :

Physical risks

These include cuts, manual handling of loads, awkward postures, falls, exposure to non-ionising radiation (laser, ultraviolet, radiofrequency) and working with machine screens. Then there are vision problems, stress and musculoskeletal problems. Ionising radiation poses a particular risk to health workers.

Noise in the workplace can lead to a risk of hearing loss, as well as cardiovascular and digestive disorders, sleep disturbances, irritability and fatigue. It also increases errors caused by carelessness.[3]

Chemical risks

These hazards play an important role in the hospital area, as health care workers can absorb chemicals when handling or being in close proximity to them. Anaesthetic gases, disinfectants, cytotoxic reagents, medicines and pharmaceutical preparations cause biological effects on workers, depending on the concentration, handling, exposure, worker sensitivity actions, exposures, triggers and protective practices adopted by employees. The use of large quantities of chemicals can cause various alterations in medical personnel, such as irritation, sensitisation processes, damage to various organs, congenital malformations, mutations and even cancer. Hazardous drugs include cytostatics or cytotoxic drugs used for cancer patients or drugs for HIV-positive patients. [3]

Biological risks

Currently, among the infectious diseases to which health professionals are exposed, bacterial aetiology stands out, such as Tuberculosis, an infectious disease caused by the bacterium Mycobacterium Tuberculosis, which affects the upper respiratory tract. This disease is common in risk groups due to its high level of exposure because of its transmission mechanism in the respiratory tract.

Psychosocial risks

Psychosocial risk factors are any condition experienced by man as he relates to his surrounding environment and the society around him in his area of work.[3]

Burnout syndrome is considered a chronic stress syndrome, the working conditions and the characteristics of the type of work performed by nurses in psychiatric, emergency and operating rooms put this group at high risk of suffering from the disease.[3]

Occupational health in the health sector in Mexico

A study conducted in a second level care hospital in Mexico showed that nursing staff in the intensive care unit are exposed to biological risks at a high level of 79%, chemical risk at a medium level 48%, physical risk at a medium level 76%, psychosocial risk at a medium level 82% and ergonomic risk at a medium level 81%. Health personnel are directly exposed to infectious diseases and contact with fluids. On the other hand, the chemical risk to which they are exposed is to substances such as cleaning products and frequent use of latex.

In terms of ergonomic risk, standing for long periods of time is the most important factor, which leads to the adoption of forced postures that cause muscular injuries. In terms of psychosocial risk, the nursing staff suffered from work-related stress and exhaustion due to physical and mental work overload.[7]

Challenges for occupational nursing in today's mexico

Mexico has systems, standards and infrastructure that promote occupational health, but despite these, it is clear that much remains to be done to ensure that workplaces can guarantee physical and emotional health and safety.

When you look at figures such as 374 million occupational accidents and 160 million occupational diseases globally, it becomes clear that the challenges are great. The ILO indicates that on average 685,000 accidents occur every day, some 475 per minute.[8]

In Mexico, the average is about 1,150 work-related accidents per day, which represents heavy costs for companies, loss of productivity and competitiveness. In the end, a public health problem.

In the short term, these figures reveal numerous challenges to be met in occupational health, including the need for greater involvement[8] , which are set out below:

Compliance with the Official Mexican Standards (NOM): In Mexico there are 43 official standards related to occupational health and safety, among which the most recent, NOM 035, stands out. In this sense, it is a challenge for companies to recognise and comply with them, but for this it is necessary to raise the quality of occupational health that goes beyond simply complying with these standards.

Adapting to changing work environments: According to the World Health Organization (WHO) workplaces, work processes and work schemes are constantly changing globally, so a major challenge is for companies to know how to adapt and be flexible in order to be able to combat the pressure, stress and work demands that are causing these constant changes.

Drug addiction care: The health of the general population in Mexico is compromised by bad habits and addictions (alcoholism, smoking), factors that must be taken into account in the workplace in order to generate measures to reverse these practices.[8]

Post-COVID era: The effects of the pandemic will continue to influence the social, economic, physical and emotional spheres for years to come. Businesses are challenged to look at this from a human perspective to ensure healthy working environments in all respects. The ILO notes that at least 25 million people will be unemployed worldwide due to COVID-19, implying an imbalance in the supply and demand for jobs. [8]

Cooperation between workers and employers: With the aim of promoting, strengthening and assimilating the modern vision of health in the workplace, in such a way as to raise awareness of the importance of occupational health.

Trained human resources: An important challenge to take into account is the need for trained human resources in occupational health, as specialised consultants are required to develop programmes, policies and actions in favour of occupational health and safety. In addition, they must be up to date on crucial issues such as the gender perspective, the fight against harassment and combating work-related stress.

Inadequate health care for workers makes socio-economic development impossible and harms more and more people. For this reason, it is a priority not only to become aware but also to act quickly, and to encourage the development of specific occupational health programmes and to strengthen existing ones. A change in corporate culture is required and, together with the managers of the organisations, to develop occupational health as an investment tool to improve productivity and profitability.[9]

In 2007, thirteen years before the pandemic, the International Council of Nurses (ICN) and the World Health Organisation (WHO) had warned that nursing professionals were in need of much stronger training to provide care and deal with the adversities that the current time demands.

There are many challenges that nurses face and will face in the spheres of care and care management, among which the following stand out: recruitment, training and sizing of specialised teams, planning of material resources, the dynamics of direct care, the lack of individual protective equipment, the precarious structure of supplements in health institutions, work overload, all situations that will require the organisation of new protocols and care flows, based on the available scientific evidence.[10]

The challenges for the future demand the need to invest in nursing to empower nurses at all levels, specifically at the most strategic levels, to ensure that they participate in high-level decision-making in health, in the design of health policies and in the functioning of health systems ensuring optimal performance of nurses to improve the satisfaction of the needs of the population they serve.[11]

In Mexico, only 7% of nurses in political leadership positions in Universities and in the Ministry of Health in Mexico have specialised training in public health, who have recently entered the field of research helping to improve governmental public health programmes.

The skills of nursing professionals in community care require data collection, analysis and presentation of data are extremely important and courses are needed in nursing schools to develop these quantitative skills covering topics such as epidemiology, economics, community assessment and informatics. However, today even nursing faculty need to be trained in these subjects; therefore, particular attention should be paid to this situation in the years to come.[12]

Challenges can be categorised as medium or long-term, depending on the estimated time frame in which they are expected to be met. However, this implies the reorientation and even the creation of policies, programmes, protocols and cross-cutting actions that, in some cases, involve various agencies and entities of the Government of the Republic, which is why it is imperative to address them so as not to go backwards or stagnate in what has been achieved in this area.[13]

Conclusions

The future of people's health care depends to a large extent on the potential of nursing work, so there is a need for trained nurses to create healthy work environment programmes, which will have an impact on providing safe and quality care.

In this sense, the occupational hazards in Mexico require the government, employers and workers to carry out preventive and protective actions that contribute to safe and hygienic companies.

Employers must provide a safe and healthy environment for their workers, which means providing access to information and training, establishing preventive measures, controlling hazards and risks, and selecting safe technology and work practices, as well as complying with occupational health legislation. [13]

Therefore, it is important to bear in mind that all workplaces are different, although the relationships and programmes under which they are regulated are similar in terms of protective measures due to the activities they carry out. The practice of occupational health nursing, if applied efficiently at the primary, secondary and tertiary levels of prevention, can lead to the development of the health, well-being, productivity and quality of life of workers for the benefit of employees, employers and society in general.[4]

While there are many challenges to mention for occupational nursing it is however necessary to highlight that skills in planning and strategy building, policy, public health advocacy and coalition building already exist in staff in some other countries, but must be strengthened to change the role of nursing, schools have an essential role to play in educating those in quantitative aspects of the essential public health functions, as these skills facilitate both individual health service delivery and population-based public health functions, thereby strengthening and empowering staff in the area of occupational health.[12]

In short, occupational nursing is in a privileged position to identify the needs of organisations within the scope of its competencies. It is for this reason that the active role it plays in its work context, its contribution is manifest in ensuring the well-being of the people it cares for, the working population. And its future lies in providing cost-effective quality care with prevention always in mind. [14]

References

1. Reyes Luna JD, Valenzuela Suazo S, Rodríguez Campo V, Reyes Luna JD, Valenzuela Suazo S, Rodríguez Campo V. Nursing in occupational health: a look at the instruments used in international research. Enfermería Actual Costa Rica [Internet]. 2019 [cited 2022 Jun 16];37(37):188-205. Available from: http://www.scielo.sa.cr/scielo.php?script=sci_arttext&pid=S1409-45682019000200188&lng=en&nrm=iso&tlng=es

2. Perez R. Challenges for health care workers in the face of coronavirus [Internet]. 2020 [cited 2022 Jun 16]. Available from: https://blogs.iadb.org/salud/es/desafios-personal-salud-coronavirus/

3. Soto L. Occupational risks of nursing staff in the infectious diseases department [Internet]. 2017 [cited 2022 Jun 16]. Available from:

https://docs.bvsalud.org/biblioref/2021/02/1148066/237.pdf

4. Juarez A. Nursing interventions in occupational health [Internet]. 2018 [cited 2022 Jun 16]. Available from: https://www.medigraphic.com/pdfs/enfermeriaimss/eim-2010/eim101e.pdf

5. Corbelle Álvarez José Manuel. La Enfermería del Trabajo, una Especialidad reciente, una Profesión de siempre. Med. Segur. trab. [Internet]. 2009 Jun [cited 2022 Sep 08]; 55(215): 10-11. Available from: http://scielo.isciii.es/scielo.php?script=sci_arttext&pid=S0465-546X2009000200001&lng=es.

6. Del M, Montelongo C, Galaviz IF. The Importance and Significance of Industrial Nursing*. 2018;

7. World Medical Association. View of Risk factors in nursing staff in a second level hospital | Ciencia Latina Revista Científica Multidisciplinar [Internet]. 2019 [cited 2022 Jun 16]. Available from: https://ciencialatina.org/index.php/cienciala/article/view/640/851

8. Occupational Health. 7 challenges of Occupational Health in Mexico [Internet]. 2018 [cited 2022 Jun 16]. Available from: https://occupationalhealth.com.mx/7-retos-de-salud-ocupacional-en-mexico/

9. Del Carmen Gastañaga M. Salud ocupacional: historia y retos del futuro occupational health: history and future challenges. Rev Peru Med Exp Salud Publica. 2019;29(2):177-8.

10. Gonzalo D. View of Nursing Challenges in times of pandemic | Science and Care Journal [Internet]. 2019 [cited 2022 Jun 16]. Available from: https://revistas.ufps.edu.co/index.php/cienciaycuidado/article/view/3134/3588

11. Moreno M. Iberoamerican Journal of Nursing Education and

Research. Build Data Capacit Patient-Centered Outcomes Res. 2022 Mar 29;

12. Pan American Health Organization. Public Health Nursing and the Essential Public Health Functions: Foundations for Professional Practice in the 21st Century. (2001) - PAHO/WHO | Pan American Health Organization [Internet]. 2020 [cited 2022 Jun 16]. Available from: https://www.paho.org/es/documentos/enfermeria-salud-publica-funciones-esenciales-salud-publica-bases-para-ejercicio-0

13. Ministry of Labour and Social Welfare. "Seguridad y Salud en el Trabajo en México: Avances, Retos y Desafíos" | Secretaría del Trabajo y Previsión Social | Gobierno | gob.mx [Internet]. 2017 [cited 2022 Jun 16]. Available from: https://www.gob.mx/stps/documentos/seguridad-y-salud-en-el-trabajo-en-mexico-avances-retos-y-desafios?idiom=es

14. González Caballero Javier. Nursing in Occupational Health, an added value for organisations. Medicine. seguro trab [Internet]. 2019 Mar [cited 2022 Sep 08] ; 65 (254): 3-9. Available from: http://scielo.isciii.es/scielo.php?script=sci_arttext&pid=S0465-546X2019000100003&lng=es. Epub 20-ene-2020. https://dx.doi.org/10.4321/s0465-546x2019000100003.

Chapter 5

Nursing, self-care and occupational health

Saying yes, just because you feel bad or guilty, will not make you the heroic nurse on the floor, it will make you a burnt out nurse in the short to medium term.

Anonymous.

Introduction

Nursing is a dynamic profession with three main focuses: promoting health and preventing illness, providing care to those who need professional assistance to achieve their optimal level of health and functioning, and research to improve the knowledge base for providing excellent nursing care.

Nursing professionals provide health care to individuals, families and communities. After assessing the client's situation and environment, the nurse identifies goals with the client, provides assistance through education and support, provides care to the client who is unable to provide care for him/herself, and interposes him/herself between the environment and the client.

This document approaches nursing from the perspective of self-care and occupational health. The contents are approached with a direction that emphasises the integral character of the concept of health in nursing workers, prevention and self-care of occupational risks that could be present in the work environment; understood as wellbeing at all levels of the life of the subjects and the positive and risky character that work has for health, as an activity that consents social life and the development of individuals in which it is unethical to put health at risk.

Work is a fundamental right of people, through which they sustain their daily lives and, of course, satisfy their basic needs and which goes beyond the physical, it is also a means by which individuals confront society, family, and even their identity. [1]

In 2004, the International Labour Organisation (ILO) called on the majority of the world's countries to seek strategies to ensure the well-being of workers and proposed solutions to "special issues", as well as to increase labour productivity, growth and well-being at work and to eliminate child labour in Latin America and the Caribbean.

The World Health Organisation (WHO) joins this important movement with its World Health Report "Working together for health", which comments on the urgent need for global concern about the health workforce crisis, especially in the poorest countries where resource shortages are even greater for health workers. [2]

Therefore, self-care is the practice of activities that people carry out in certain periods of time for themselves and in the interest of maintaining a healthy work, as well as continuing personal development and well-being by satisfying requirements for functional and developmental regulations, as well as being an action of autonomy.

Nursing has the main function of health care, which together with the health team is responsible for promoting the self-care of people, who should not only develop actions for the promotion of health, but should also show in their person, healthy habits practices for self-care in health institutions and with them be able to provide a quality service and wellbeing for both individuals.[3]

It is important to mention that nursing staff are exposed to multiple risks and factors that could seriously affect their health, when carrying out activities in which they do not have sufficient material or do not have self-care and safety habits, in addition to other attitudes that end up affecting their work performance, all of which could be avoided with the corresponding self-care and established prevention actions, a practice that is sometimes not carried out due to the multiple roles that nursing professionals fulfil, putting their health at risk.

The self-care of the health of nursing staff is the argument of importance of this research, nursing staff as health professionals interact in society and participate as active members in it, as they have a solid training based on technical, scientific, humanistic and ethical foundations that allow them to carry out their practice with responsibility and quality.

Occupational health and occupational hazards

To begin this section it is necessary to recapitulate the conceptualization of self-care, for its part the World Health Organization defines self-care as synonymous with self-care, it is defined as "the ability of individuals, families and communities to promote health, prevent disease, maintain health and cope with illness and disability with or without the support of a health professional", it is considered as the main subject of action for the care and prevention of oneself (whether an individual or a community), giving great importance to the actions taken by individuals for this care. [4]. The idea of self-care should not only be promoted, but should also be exclusively linked to people outside the health area, as it is a reality that all health personnel are highly predisposed to a diversity of illnesses and/or accidents caused by the characteristics of the area itself. This goes hand in hand with another concept, which is occupational health, defined as the set of activities that promote the comfort of workers, thus preventing work-related illnesses. But why is it relevant? Because the working class is part of the basis for the proper functioning of society; comparing it with the way it exists in health institutions, we can say that nursing is part of that basis of utmost importance for the proper functioning of health systems. [5]

Data from the International Labour Organization (ILO) indicate that deaths from occupational diseases in 2017 were 2.7 million; while the Pan American Health Organization (PAHO) shows that in Latin America only 1% to 5% of occupational diseases are reported. These small but shocking figures reveal the situation that working people experience on a daily basis. Now, with regard to the area of health, the Organisation for Economic Co-operation and Development (OECD), published the health outlook for Mexico in 2021, which shows that the country occupies one of the lowest positions with regard to the number-ratio of nursing staff-patients, where the other OECD countries have around 9 nurses per 1,000 inhabitants, while Mexico has a ratio of 3 nurses per 1,000 inhabitants. [6] These data show a reality where the Mexican health system finds itself with a large amount of demand, but few professionals to meet it; during the COVID-19 pandemic, a side that was not visible to many was revealed: the lack of working conditions for nurses in the hospital area. [7] Working conditions, work overload, hostility in the hospital, requirement for further updates, emotional exhaustion, shortage of equipment, little emotional support: the perception of nurses regarding their working conditions. And it is not only these factors that promote occupational diseases, but there is also the presence of occupational hazards, which can be defined as any event that can endanger both workers and employers in a company, causing physical or psychological harm. [8]

Nursing and the concept of self-care

Self-care is aimed at the practice of activities that people, who want to, can do according to their temporary situation and on their own, in order to live well, maintain and/or regain health and prolong life.

In this sense, Orem's General Theory of Self-Care Deficit points out the importance of its application in the development of nursing knowledge, in addition to its great usefulness for the training of human resources and nursing practice; the role currently occupied by nursing in the disciplines of the health area and in society is determined by its trajectory and work over the course of time, influenced by a series of facts and circumstances that have defined its actions and its social function.

It is well known that nurses are constantly confronted with life-threatening risks due to their work which exposes them to situations or activities. Therefore, nursing professionals are not exempt from such occupational hazards, which can be related to contact with diseases and an unsafe working environment, biological, chemical or physical factors. It is therefore important to have basic and specialised protective equipment according to the area of work.

There are a large number of risks to workers' health in the working environment. Risk factors are defined as the physical, chemical, biological and social elements or phenomena that can constitute a risk to the health of workers by deteriorating it and which, directly or indirectly, are related to work, manifesting themselves in the form of injuries, occupational diseases, pathologies and other health imbalances.

Let's start by talking about some of the key terms in the chapter that should be known for a better understanding. The working environment is understood as the set of conditions that surround the working person and that, directly or indirectly, influence his or her health and life. The work environment is the place where the factors that damage and pollute the environment inside and outside the company are generated. [2]

Nursing self-care in occupational diseases

As previously mentioned, self-care is defined as the practice of activities that people carry out in certain periods of time for themselves and with the interest of maintaining a healthy work, as well as continuing with personal development and wellbeing by satisfying requirements for functional and developmental regulations, as well as being an action of autonomy; this term determines the existence of the work that each individual carries out to perpetuate that health that is so much desired in times of crisis. Nursing has dedicated itself year after year to the promotion and dissemination of this concept, being a fundamental part of the work carried out by the staff, but many times, it is forgotten that the best way to promote something is by doing it oneself; knowing, knowing and practising in order to find out what the benefit is.

The previous point was about occupational risks in occupational health, as nursing is one of those sciences that is exposed to a large number of risk factors, both biological and physical, as well as psychosocial and social. So all this has an end, like everything else: occupational illness.

The Mexican Social Security Institute (IMSS) presents reports to clarify information about the occupational health of employees (be they nurses, doctors, therapists, etc.), providing information about a variety of occupational health issues. For this chapter, information about occupational diseases registered during the year 2020 will be used. Information about 119 474 persons was collected, where health personnel accounted for 90% (108 325). But for reasons, only the numbers of nursing staff will be used.

Total national	Nurses (technical)	Specialist nurses	Nursing assistants
108 325	19 018	13 724	5 692

The data presented here gives us an approximation of the number of staff in the institution, but it also gives us an idea of the occupational illnesses that have most afflicted these staff. According to the IMSS data, the 10 most common illnesses in 2020 were [3]:

Occupational disease	Technical nurses	Specialist nurses	Nursing assistants
COVID-19	18 701	13 510	10 856
Infectious and parasitic diseases	179	147	116

	24	18	6
Respiratory diseases associated with COVID-19	24	18	6
Contact dermatitis	23	11	8
Carpal tunnel syndrome	6	1	--
Eye disease and its annexes	4	3	3
Mental and behavioural disorders	3	1	1
Dorsopathies	1	1	--
Shoulder injuries	2	--	--
Radial styloid tenosynovitis of (Quervain)	2	3	1

Self-care in the face of COVID-19

Originated in Wuhan, China, giving its first outbreak in December 2019 and being considered pandemic on March 11, 2020, SARS-CoV-2 is a virus of the order *Nidovirales* and the family *Coronaviridae, is* characterized by being enveloped, pleomorphic or spherical, which present RNA as genome and whose size ranges from 80 to 120 nm in diameter; producing the disease that is COVID-19, characterized by the presence cough, dyspnea, fever, headache, among others. [9]. In the case of Mexico, for the year 2021, a total of 283, 122 cases were re-exported among health personnel; where nursing personnel presented the greatest number of cases with 38.9% (110, 134 cases), and in the case of deaths, there were a total of 4, 517 and nursing personnel presented a total of 858 deaths. [10].

It is therefore necessary for nursing staff to ask themselves, what actions should they take to combat these figures? The first line for this self-care is information and training in the situation; as a result, in 2019 the "Strategic Nursing Response Plan to covid-19" was generated by the Standing Commission on Nursing (CPE) and meetings with the heads of the State Nursing Coordinating Bodies, where the entry to training in COVID-19 is allowed, and important points are addressed such as: care interventions for frontline health personnel; use of personal protective equipment; person (patient) centred care; response to assaults on health personnel; interventions by nursing students. Its impact was such that several virtual courses for continuing nursing education were generated, such as the course on "Correct use of Personal Protective Equipment". Similarly, this is only the physical and biological side, but it should also be noted the relevance there is for the proper care of mental health in nursing; it has always been a reality that nursing suffers from a great mental burden, but with the emergence of the pandemic, these concerns were enhanced and exposed. According to the survey "Fears and concerns of health personnel in relation to covid-19: elaboration, validation and application of a survey", more than 90% of respondents showed a fear of contagion and of transmitting the disease to their loved ones, such is the fear of such an event that 88% had had psychosomatic symptoms related to the coronavirus. Similarly, more than 80% were concerned about the shortage of personal protective equipment and even about the lack of support received by the institutions about the possibilities of becoming infected; similarly, a hard side of fear and uncertainty is manifested, 85% of them presented a great concern regarding discrimination and harassment that they could receive for being part of the health team. [11]

Self-care of infectious and parasitic diseases

Both infectious and parasitic diseases can be defined, or summarised, as all those pathologies/disorders caused by any organism, whether bacterial, virulent, fungal or parasitic in nature. The impact of this type of disease is of great relevance, as they are one of the main causes of illness in children and older adults, all caused by situations of poor hygiene. For 2016, the Juarez Hospital indicated that the most common parasitic diseases were amebiasis with 47 thousand cases and giardiasis with 2 thousand. It can be seen that the main reason for infectious diseases is poor hygiene, and compared to self-care, there is a deficiency in the prevention of such situations.[12]

With regard to nursing, there is a great responsibility for the care of patients and for oneself; this is so important that the Centre for Disease Control and Prevention (CDC) has created committees for the detection, approach and application of basic practices for the good control and prevention of infectious diseases. These are present in two aspects, actions taken by managers and actions taken by nursing staff; the first consists of four points, which summarises: the heads of nursing, together with the other managers, must ensure that the necessary resources are provided so that the frontline staff can carry out their practices without becoming infected; there must be constant education and training for the staff, where not only the information acquired must be shown, but also demonstrated in practice; the nursing staff must be well informed in order to be able to carry out their practices without becoming infected; nursing should be well informed in order to give back to the community, promoting education and self-care to others, be they family members, patients or even co-workers; and the existence of performance monitoring, noting how this education itself promotes prevention or not. Then the standard nursing precautions for infectious diseases are presented, which will promote practices that will prevent the movement of pathogens, both nurse-patient and patient-nurse; the first is the most basic practice of a person in the health area: proper hand washing; it follows that proper cleaning and disinfection of the workplace is a key component in preventing contact transmission; safety in infections and medications, where it is identified that the necessary materials must be provided to be able to carry out care (medication administration) in the safest way, due to the existence of infectious outbreaks caused by unsafe practices such as the reuse of syringes, insulin injectors, among others; application of sanitary protocols to minimise potential exposures, such as the use of PPE, cough protocols, hand hygiene, among others.

Self-care in the face of mental illness and disorders

Mental health is referred to as a state of well-being whereby individuals recognise their abilities and are able to cope with the normal stresses of life. Considering that nursing is a science primarily concerned with the health care of a variety of people, stress is something that is normally experienced, to such an extent that the mental workload is of a high level. This mental load, subject to the definition of the set of psychophysical requirements to which a person is subjected during their working day; if it is transported to nursing, we observe how this branch of the health sciences comes up against a diversity of obstacles that increase this mental load, from the empathy they feel towards their patients, the bad treatment they may receive from patients/family members, the scarcity of resources, exposure to illnesses, shifts of more than 12 hours, among others, cause a high level of mental exhaustion. This has reached a point where the use of psychoactive substances has become normalised as a method to suffocate and reduce this burden, where a study carried out in Bogotá determined that nursing staff use alcohol, cigarettes and energy drinks, and it was also determined that they also use barbiturates, antidepressants, amphetamines and opiates. And these long-standing issues were exploited by the pandemic, revealing the reality in which many staff have suffered for years. [13]

The World Health Organisation has made a number of recommendations for the management of stressful situations for health workers, including: identifying tools for the correct management of stress, almost as soon as you have one, you should proceed to maintain it; allowing the normalisation of feelings, sharing feelings among colleagues; taking care of basic needs; avoiding the use of unhealthy strategies such as alcohol consumption, smoking and drug use. [14] Other types of care have been identified following the global situation with regard to COVID-19. Physical activity has been one of the main drivers for change and improvement of the mental health situation, the study "*The need to maintain regular physical activity while taing precautions*" where it states that due to person to person distancing caused a decrease in physical activity, and with quarantine, This is why basic and safe activities are recommended (and that can be done at home), promoting not only the appearance of metabolic diseases but also increasing mental satiety, where mental health is viscerally related to physical health. Another of the recommendations is the practice of *mindfulness*, where the study "*Relationships between midnfulness practice and levels of midndfulness, medical and psychological symptmos and well-being a mindfulness-based stress reduction program*" where it is possible to visualise how this technique allows people who live under constant anxiety and stress to disconnect and leave aside work life and get closer to a peace of mind, after leaving intrusive thoughts that generate greater stress.

Conclusions

As evidenced in there are various situations and measures that health personnel should put into practice for self-care in their work, emphasising the importance of this, as well as mentioning the established measures or health protocols that should be taken into account when carrying out work activities. Therefore, self-care is focused on health promotion as a way of building a healthy life, which contributes basic components to healthy lifestyles and work, which go beyond strengthening or changing people's lifestyles and ways of acting, in order to put into practice behaviours that enhance safety and health.

In conclusion, occupational health and healthy work environments are among the most precious assets of individuals, communities and countries. A healthy work environment is indispensable, not only for the health of workers, but also for making a positive contribution to productivity, work motivation, work spirit, job satisfaction and overall quality of life.

While it is true that self-care has been studied by different disciplinary and professional fields, it must be approached in an interdisciplinary way, which is why occupational health and safety is involved in an approach where the worker is studied holistically and his or her health is analysed as the result of the care that each individual provides for him or herself, of his or her ability to make decisions, to control life and to ensure that society offers all its members the possibility of enjoying a good state of health.

References

1. Luna JDR. scielo. [Online]; 2019. Accessed June 18, 2022. Available from: https://www.scielo.sa.cr/pdf/enfermeria/n37/1409-4568-enfermeria-37-188.pdf.

2. SCd. istas training. [Online]; 2015. Accessed 14 June 2022. Available from: istas.

Garduño-Santo A. uaemex. [Online]; 2017. Accessed 15 June 2022. Available at: http://web.uaemex.mx/revistahorizontes/docs/revistas/Vol5/2_AUTOCUIDADO.pdf.

4. OMdl Health. who. [Online]; 2022. Accessed June 17, 2022. Available from: https://www.who.int/es/health-topics/self-care#tab=tab_1.

5. Mino O. journals.usat. [Online]; 2019. Accessed June 18, 2022. Available from: https://revistas.usat.edu.pe/index.php/cietna/article/view/251/909.

6. Glance Haa. oecd.org. [Online]; 2021. Accessed 18 June 2022. Available from: https://www.oecd.org/centrodemexico/medios/NOTA%20DE%20PAIS%20MEXICO.pdf.

7. Quintana MO. scielo. [Online]; 2021. Accessed 14 June 2022. Available at: http://www.scielo.org.mx/scielo.php?pid=S2448-60942020000400003&script=sci_arttext.

8. UNIR. [Online]; 2021. Accessed 14 June 2022. Available at: https://ecuador.unir.net/actualidad-unir/riesgos-laborales/.

9. Salud Sdl. gob.mx. [Online]; 2022. Accessed 15 June 2022. Available from: https://coronavirus.gob.mx/wp-content/uploads/2022/01/2022.01.12-Lineamiento_VE_ERV_DGE.pdf.

10. Health sdl. gob.mx. [Online]; 2022. Accessed June 16, 2022. Available from: https://www.gob.mx/cms/uploads/attachment/file/678408/PERSONALDESALUD_25.10.21.pdf.

11. Grajales RAZ. aladefe. [Online]; 2020. Accessed June 16, 2022. Available at: https://www.aladefe.org/noticias/Enfermeria_y_Covid.pdf.

12. WHO. gob.mx. [Online]; 2019. Accessed June 15, 2022. Available from: https://www.gob.mx/salud/prensa/162-ninos-y-adultos-mayores-principales-afectados-por-la-parasitosis#:~:text=Inform%C3%B3%20that%20in%20M%20C3%A9xico%20las,dos%20mil%20de%20la%20la%20segunda.

13. Zambrano CLM. Scielo. [Online]; 2017. Accessed 15 June 2022. Available from: https://www.scielo.cl/scielo.php?script=sci_arttext&pid=S0717-95532015000100005.

14. Ferran MB. Pub Med central. [Online]; 2021. Accessed June 16, 2022. Available at: https://www.ncbi.nlm.nih.gov/pmc/articles/PMC7229967/.

II. GENDER-BASED VIOLENCE AND BREASTFEEDING

Chapter 6

Prevention, care and eradication of violence against women in the workplace

Violence creates more social problems than it solves.

Martin Luther King

Introduction

This chapter addresses the issue of workplace violence, with the aim of making it visible, informing and raising awareness among nursing professionals about the problem, as well as highlighting strategies for its prevention and eradication. The generalities, main concepts and international and national statistics on the subject are presented. In this way, as a first point, it is recognised that working is the fundamental axis of the human being, which allows people to achieve a different standard of living. Work is a human right in itself, inherent to people, so the state is obliged to guarantee the best conditions so that everyone can exercise it with dignity, in equal conditions and without any restriction or discrimination. [1]

In the workplace, however, violence as an act is present in workplaces and other centres of concentration of people, and it is so present that it is often perceived as an inescapable component of the human condition. [2]

Specifically talking about workplace violence, harassment and sexual harassment in the work environment are behaviours that affect people's self-esteem and work performance. The result is a series of psychological and physical effects that lead to discomfort; however, this is an overlooked and unclear procedure, which will only bring legal uncertainty to both parties and will not solve the underlying problem. It is therefore important to know how to deal with violence, harassment and sexual harassment in the workplace, so that victims and legal agencies can act to protect the free development of the personality and the physical and psychological well-being of employees. [3]

In this regard, the International Labour Organisation (ILO), of which Mexico is a member, at its 108th General Conference held in Geneva on 10 June 2019, recognised the right of everyone to work free of violence and harassment, including gender-based violence and harassment. (4) However, historically, women and men have participated differently in all areas of life and the gender division of labour has had an unequal impact on opportunities, especially for women. [1]

In this sense, the following chapter sets out guidelines for the prevention of and attention to violence and may also be a useful instrument for raising awareness among public servants, as it includes general aspects of the topic, explaining the meaning of violence, workplace violence, workplace harassment and sexual harassment. It also mentions statistics related to the topic, prevention measures and the process of care in case of workplace violence.

General aspects

According to the World Health Organisation (WHO) violence is the intentional use of physical force, threats against oneself, another person, a group or a community that results in or is likely to result in trauma, psychological harm, developmental problems or death. [5]

According to the General Law on Women's Access to a Life Free of Violence (LGAMVLLV), Article 10 defines workplace violence, including sexual harassment and stalking, as types of such violence: [2]

"It is exercised by persons who have an employment relationship, regardless of the hierarchical relationship, consisting of an act or omission in abuse of power that damages the self-esteem, health, integrity, freedom and security of the victim, and impedes their development and violates equality. It may consist of a single harmful event or a series of events, the sum of which produces the harm. It is worth mentioning that it includes a number of related elements such as sexual harassment, harassment at work and sexual harassment. [2]

Both sexual harassment and sexual harassment are expressed in verbal or physical conduct, or both, related to sexuality or for lewd purposes. While in sexual harassment there is an abusive exercise of power that leads to a state of defencelessness and risk for the victim, regardless of whether it is carried out in one or more elements, in sexual harassment, on the other hand, there is an exercise of power, in a relationship of real subordination of the victim to the aggressor in the workplace.

Similarly, workplace bullying addresses a series of events that are intended to cause physical, psychological, economic, occupational and professional harm by intimidating, excluding, dulling, flattening, or emotionally or intellectually consuming the victim. (2) It is worth mentioning that workplace bullying can be represented mainly in three ways: upward, horizontal and downward. Upward bullying refers to the existence of an individual holding a higher hierarchical rank in the organisation, who is assaulted by one or more subordinates. On the other hand, horizontal harassment is that in which a worker is harassed by a colleague with the same hierarchical level and finally, downward harassment is a behaviour in which the person who holds the power through contempt, false accusations, and even insults, aims to undermine the psychological environment of the harassed worker in order to stand out from his/her subordinates, to maintain his/her hierarchical position, or it is simply a business strategy whose objective is to get rid of a specific person by forcing him/her to leave "voluntarily" without legally dismissing him/her, as this would entail an economic cost for the company without any reason. [1]

Among our human rights is the right to work, the main characteristic of which is respect for the dignity of people, and for this reason we promote the right to live in a work environment free of violence, which guarantees equity, substantive equality and the right to non-discrimination.

In order to emphasise the importance of this right, the ILO pointed out that decent work:

"It synthesises people's aspirations during their working lives, and means the opportunity to access productive employment that generates a fair income, security in the workplace and social protection for families, better prospects for personal development and social integration, freedom for individuals to express their views, organise and participate in the decisions that affect their lives, and equality of opportunity and treatment for all, women and men".

It is important to emphasise the different and probable sources of workplace violence, which may include stress factors, whether personal, occupational, economic or social. In the workplace, stress is a general and common response to risk factors, which can lead to people or workers becoming aggressive to a certain extent in the face of a high level of stress in their lives.

Despite this, the most commonly heard and known cases of workplace violence are mainly related to two elements: gender inequality and abuse of power.

In the first element, workplace violence is more associated with the inequity and inequality that exists between the two sexes, with the result that, traditionally, men are the ones who should and have held most of the positions of power. This demonstrates that gender equality considerations are deeply rooted in the power relations that prevail in the world of work, with an abysmal imbalance, mostly favouring men.

In the second element, due to the existence of hierarchy in institutions, companies or organisations, the abuse of power can become normalised and in this respect the ILO stated that: "Traditionally, authority and the exercise of control over others in the workplace have been regarded as legitimate forms of power, since they derive more from the positions people hold in an organisation than from the individuals themselves". However, it is always necessary to identify elements that may cross the boundary between what is and is not tolerable and what is and is not allowed in workplace relationships and that could trigger some form of workplace violence.

As mentioned above, violence implies a power relationship in which the perpetrator of violence has the legitimate power of domination. In labour relations are hierarchical in nature, violence at work is initially exercised by those who are in a better position in the hierarchy, although it is not uncommon that it is also carried out by peers and possibly subordinates. [6]

Zarpf, Knors and Kulla refer to seven areas in which bullying or harassment at work takes place: [6]

- Organisational measures, such as assigning tasks that are not the person's responsibility
- Social isolation, e.g. separating the person from the group, not inviting them to meetings or activities that take place in the office.
- Attacks on the person's private life, e.g. making critical remarks about family or partner
- Physical violence, i.e. pulling, pushing, shoving, hitting, etc.
- Attacks on a person's beliefs or conditions, e.g. religious beliefs or physical characteristics
- Verbal aggression, such as name-calling and shouting
- Rumours that discredit people.

Both women and men suffer from the above conditions and behaviours, but to varying degrees. In the case of women, the unequal power relationship they have with men in society as a whole, in the workplace, means that they suffer violence not only from people who are their hierarchical superiors, but also from their peers, subordinates, and sometimes even from people outside the workplace (users, clients or suppliers of goods or services).

This is evidenced by statistics where in the case of Mexico, the working population amounts to 55.7 million people, of which 39% are women who at some point have experienced an atmosphere of violence against them, both horizontally and vertically. In this context, the National Human Rights Commission (CNDH) prepared a document entitled "Diagnosis of sexual harassment and sexual harassment in the federal public administration 2015-2018", which revealed that of 402 victims who reported harassment and abuse in institutions, 94.53% were women, 3.23% were men and in 2.24% of cases the sex of the victim was not indicated. [7]

In the same vein, the National Institute of Statistics and Geography (INEGI), through the National Survey on the Dynamics of Household Relationships (ENDIREH), showed that 26.6% of women who work or have ever worked have experienced some violent act in the workplace, mainly of a sexual or discriminatory nature by their work colleagues (sexual harassment at work) with 35.2%, followed by their superiors (sexual harassment at work) with 19.3%. Regarding the type of aggression, 47.9% was sexual, 3.7% was physical and 48.9% was emotional. As for the place where the violence occurred, 79.1% took place on work premises and 11.5% in a public place close to work. [8]

This does not mean that men do not experience violence and harassment, but that statistics show that these behaviours are higher in relation to women.

Preventive measures in situations of workplace violence

For the purpose of this document, prevention will be understood as all those activities, actions or initiatives aimed at anticipating, detecting in a timely manner and preventing acts or conduct of harassment and sexual and/or workplace harassment in the public entities of the state government with the objective of eliminating the number of cases of workplace violence and thereby protecting the right of individuals to a life free of violence and/or harassment. [9]

The responsibility for the supervision and continuous monitoring of work environments lies with the institution where the workers are employed. This makes it possible to verify in a systematic and timely manner whether conditions or expressions of harassment and sexual and workplace harassment are present in the environment, as well as their magnitude and seriousness, in order to design the best strategies for their elimination. [9]

The actions that need to be taken to this end are the elaboration of diagnoses or surveys on the incidence and seriousness of the problem applied periodically and with reliable methodologies, as well as active surveillance activities by key actors trained to identify signs of harassment or sexual harassment and workplace violence in the environment, such as a hostile environment, sexist or discriminatory images, messages that reproduce stereotypes or discriminatory content, among others. [9]

All prevention actions should aim to promote a culture of respect for the integrity and human and labour rights of all staff and to discourage the incidence of violent or discriminatory behaviour. Therefore, the best form of prevention will always be to promote positive working relationships and respect for the autonomy, dignity and human rights of all people; such conditions make violence less likely to occur. [10]

Other preventive measures that can be mentioned are the following: [10]

- Provide visibility and recognition of the importance of addressing the problem of gender-based violence in the workplace by publicly and consciously involving women in certain decision-making positions; while this alone does not guarantee that problems of violence or discrimination will disappear, it sends a clear message that the company/agency intends to promote equal participation.

- Establish an area responsible for dealing with petitions or requests for intervention so that workers have a space for conciliation and remedy when the situation does not compromise their wellbeing, as well as for guidance, accompaniment and denunciation when the aggressions transgress criminal, civil or labour laws that affect their rights and interests.

- Creation or adoption of an internal route or model protocol for dealing with these situations, followed by actions for its implementation in the company, body or agency, including the determination of the areas in charge of its application, monitoring and imposition of sanctions; the persons assigned and the person in charge, the stages of the procedure to be followed and its duration, as well as the rules to be followed to prove the existence of the accusations.

- Companies, bodies or agencies that may have a public or authoritative character are subject to specific and delimited obligations in relation to the conduct of an investigation and due process to resolve the situation of violence experienced by a person, to ensure their integrity and to resolve the investigation within a reasonable time in order to sanction the persons responsible.

Process of care in the event of workplace violence

The objective of this route is to establish the necessary actions to address cases of alleged workplace violence, harassment and sexual harassment, with the aim of protecting the dignity and integrity of workers, through a clear and precise scheme that inhibits the commission of such practices and provides advice to complainants or complainants during the processes of access to justice. [9]

In dealing with cases of workplace violence, including workplace harassment, sexual harassment and sexual harassment in the workplace, the alleged victim should be informed of the existence of different avenues for resolving the case: [2]

- Workplace, through the same counsellor and/or the Care and Follow-up Committee.
- PROFEDET.
- Conciliation Centres.
- Labour Courts.

Similarly, the alleged victim should be reminded that the proceedings under the Protocol do not limit his or her right to initiate proceedings through other jurisdictional channels such as civil or criminal.

Eradicating workplace violence

The International Labour Conference was an important element in the adoption of the ILO's Centenary Declaration on the Future of Work, which expressed a clear commitment to promote a world of work free from violence and harassment. In the framework of this Conference, the commitment was made concrete through the adoption of Convention 190 on violence and harassment, the first international treaty establishing the right to a world of work free from violence and harassment and regulating a common and clear framework to prevent and address violence and harassment in an inclusive and gender-sensitive approach. [11]

In terms of the specific obligations that ratifying states must fulfil, they commit themselves, among others, to a number of key elements for eradication: [11]

- Ensure working environments free of violence and harassment.
- Developing comprehensive policies to prevent and combat violence and harassment
- Integrate definitions of harassment and violence at work, including gender-based violence and harassment, into national legislation.
- Establish appropriate and effective remedies and redress in cases of harassment and violence at work.
- Determine grievance and investigation procedures and resolution mechanisms within and outside the workplace.
- Implement a system of labour inspections by state agencies empowered to issue orders for immediate action or the interruption of work in cases of imminent danger to the life, health, integrity or safety of workers.
- Determine measures to ensure the protection of complainants, victims, witnesses and whistleblowers in cases of workplace violence and harassment.
- Require through domestic legislation that employers devise appropriate measures commensurate with their degree of control to prevent workplace violence and harassment.

In order to efficiently interpret the Convention, the ILO adopted Recommendation 206 on violence and harassment in the world of work. Among the main recommendations that help to better interpret the obligations contained in the Convention are the following: [11]

Definitions of violence and harassment in the world of work should be incorporated into the labour and employment, occupational safety and health, equality and non-discrimination and criminal law of States ratifying the Convention, as appropriate.

- Internal regulations should define the rights and obligations of workers and the employer. It also stresses the need to take into account factors that increase the likelihood of violence and harassment, including psychosocial hazards and risks. Appropriate measures should be taken for sectors or occupations and work patterns most exposed to violence and harassment, such as night work, work performed in isolation, work in the health sector, hospitality, social services, emergency services, domestic work, transport, education and leisure.
- With regard to remedies and reparations, States should implement measures such as: the right to resign from the employment relationship; compensation; reinstatement of the worker; appropriate compensation for resulting damages; immediate enforcement orders to ensure that certain behaviours are stopped or to require changes in policies or practices; payment of legal fees and costs; compensation in case of injury or illness of a psychosocial, physical or any other nature, resulting in an inability to work.
- For complaints and conflict resolution, measures to be implemented should include: establishment of courts with staff specialised in gender-based violence and harassment issues; prompt and efficient handling of cases; legal assistance and counselling for complainants and victims.

- Establish counselling services or other measures for perpetrators of violence and harassment in the world of work in order to prevent reoffending and, where appropriate, facilitate their return to work.

This has an impact not only on domestic labour law but also on civil, administrative and criminal law, as it should not be forgotten that harassment or bullying should be classified as a criminal offence under domestic law.

Conclusions

It is significant to mention the importance, relevance and impact that this issue confers, since nowadays, multiple cases of violence, discrimination and harassment have been seen in the workplace, and derived from this, it is important to know the damage in the physical and mental well-being that can be caused in workers who suffer from workplace violence, which is why the prevention, attention and eradication of it, should be an intrinsic and fundamental issue for companies, both private and public, since, with this, great advances can be achieved in terms of the issue.

To learn about workers' rights, as well as the protocol for the prevention, attention and eradication of situations of violence, discrimination or harassment of workers in a company.

By encouraging the implementation of such a protocol against workplace violence in the various companies in the country and in the world, it helps to reduce the number of cases of such situations, which not only implies a growth in a healthy working environment in the company, but also a growth in a professional way, as this would indicate an increase in the well-being of workers and thus the production and effectiveness of the company.

On the other hand, it is of utmost relevance that in the workplace these aspects related to workplace violence are taken more seriously, where actions that lead to a better coexistence at work are gradually reinforced. Similarly, it is essential that the institution has complete and reliable information on workplace harassment, including sexual harassment, as this will help to strengthen the diagnosis of this problem in order to design strategies for prevention, attention, investigation and, where appropriate, punishment of conduct that constitutes workplace harassment and sexual harassment, applicable at public and private level, with the aim of achieving a violence-free working environment.

References

1. Carmona Midl. Guidelines for the prevention, care and eradication of workplace violence. [Online]; 2020. Accessed 15 June 2022. Available at: http://www.congresochihuahua2.gob.mx/descargas/finanzas/contabilida d5/12293.pdf.

2. Ministry of Labour and Social Security. Protoloco para prevenir, atender y erradicar la violencia laboral en los centros de trabajo. [Online]; 2020. Accessed 15 June 2022. Available at: https://www.gob.mx/cms/uploads/attachment/file/539287/Protocolo_Viol encia_Laboral_0603-1amGMX__1_.pdf.

3. General Directorate of Attention to Women in Guanajuato. Protocolo para prevenir y atender la violencia laboral, el hostigamiento y acoso sexual. [Online]; 2020. Accessed June 15, 2022. Available at: http://www.guanajuatocapital.gob.mx/files/2019-09/Protocolo%20para%20Prevenir%20y%20Atender%20la%20Violencia %20Laboral,%20Hostigamiento%20y%20Acoso%20Sexual.pdf.

4. Banxico. Protocol for the prevention, attention and sanction of cases of labour violence and discrimination in the bank of mexico. [Online].; 2019. Accessed June 15, 2022. Available from: http://transparencia.banxico.org.mx/documentos/%7BA6302BBC-32E0-E974-0AD8-B1F0AD15E67D%7D.pdf.

5. World Health Organisation (WHO). Violence. [Online]; 2018. Accessed 15 June 2022. Available from: http://www.who.int/topics/violence/es/...

6. Government of the State of Guanajuato. Protocol to prevent and address workplace violence, harassment and sexual harassment.

[Online]; 2017. Accessed 15 June 2022. Available from: https://www.codegto.gob.mx/wp-content/uploads/2017/01/PROTOCOLO-PAVLAHSGto.pdf.

7. National Human Rights Commission. Diagnosis of sexual harassment and sexual harassment in the federal public administration 2015-2018. [Online]; 2019. Accessed 28 June 2022. Available from: https://igualdaddegenero.cndh.org.mx/Content/doc/Publicaciones/Diagn ostico-HostigamientoAcoso-Sexual-APF.pdf. Accessed 20/10/2020 at 14:10.

8. National Institute of Statistics and Geography (INEGI). Encuenta nacional sobre la dinámica de las relaciones en los hogares. [Online]; 2017. Accessed 28 June 2022. Available from: https://www.inegi.org.mx/programas/endireh/2016/.

9. Instituto Tecnologico Superior del Sur de Guanajuato. Protocol to prevent and address workplace violence, harassment and sexual harassment at the instituto tecnologico superior del sur de guanajuato. [Online].; 2019. Accessed 28 June 2022. Available from: http://www.itsur.edu.mx/documentos_publicados/estadistica/politica_igu aldad_laboral_y_no_discriminacion/Protocolo_para_prevenir_y_atender _VLAHS_en_el_ITSUR.pdf.

10. United Nations Office on Drugs and Crime (UNODC). General guidelines on gender-based violence in the workplace for workplaces in Mexico. [Online]; 2019. Accessed 28 June 2022. Available from: https://www.unodc.org/documents/mexicoandcentralamerica/2020/Mexic o/Lineamientos_generales_sobre_violencia_de_genero_en_el_ambito_l aboral_para_los_centros_de_trabajo_en_Mexico.pdf.

11. International Labour Organization (ILO). Eliminating violence and harassment in the world of work. Convention 190, Recommendation 206 and accompanying Resolution. [Online]; 2019. Accessed 28 June 2022. Available from: https://www.ilo.org/wcmsp5/groups/public/---dgreports/---dcomm/---publ/documents/meetingdocument/wcms_721395.pdf.

Chapter 7

Breastfeeding rooms, set-up and operation

The social norms associated with the ideal defining "intensive motherhood" suggest a one-to-one relationship along the lines of "working mother=neglected childhood" and "working mother=neglected childhood".

Mª del C. Rodríguez.

Introduction

Breastfeeding is the optimal way to feed babies, providing the nutrients they need in a balanced way, while protecting against morbidity and mortality due to infectious diseases (PAHO).

In this respect, the National Institute of Statistics and Geography (INEGI) reported that 19.9 million women work in a paid activity during the year. Of these, 14.7 million are mothers, representing 73.86 per cent of employed women in Mexico.

Today many women are part of the labour force in Mexico, and a percentage of them have chosen to become mothers, so the federal labour law must guarantee the exercise of the right to breastfeed, i.e. they must receive information and timely guidance as established by the National Human Rights Commission.

When talking about breastfeeding, not only the benefits for the newborn are highlighted, but also the benefits for the mother's health and the promotion of attachment, thus ensuring comprehensive care for the mother-child pair.

Therefore, it is important that governmental programmes and laws are developed in favour of working mothers, as well as the creation of quality spaces to carry out the breastfeeding process without affecting their working day, demonstrating that women can be immersed in several roles at the same time with the support of laws that allow for their personal and professional growth.

Background on breastfeeding

The current recommendation of the World Health Organisation is that the newborn should be exclusively breastfed from the first hour of birth until 6 months of age, at which time complementary feeding with other age-appropriate foods and fluids is initiated and continued until 24 months of age, or longer if both mother and child so desire. [1]

In Mexico, evidence indicates that over time there has been an alarming deterioration in breastfeeding practices, with the lowest rates of exclusive breastfeeding in children under 6 months of age in continental America. National studies indicate that barriers to breastfeeding range from those of an individual nature to those related to the socio-cultural environment and policies in the country.

Since the 1970s, international organisations such as the United Nations Children's Fund (UNICEF) and the World Health Organisation (WHO) have been working to improve breastfeeding rates; thanks to these efforts, the International Labour Organisation (ILO), Mexico began to make changes to the regulatory and public policy framework until the creation of the National Breastfeeding Committee in 1995, which underwent significant changes from its establishment until its disappearance when it was incorporated into the National Committee of the Even Start in Life Programme.

On the other hand, the Constitution of the United Mexican States, the Federal Labour Law, the laws of the Social Security Institutes, the Mexican Standards, among others, have been reformed to protect breastfeeding mothers in the workplace. This has been done in order to encourage working women to breastfeed through the creation of breastfeeding breaks or reduced working hours, maternity leave, and the employer's obligation to provide mothers with a hygienic place to feed their children or express breast milk (breastfeeding facilities).

However, many Mexican companies do not have the aforementioned facilities, or worse still do not grant full permits or licences, which may be due to the lack of sanctions for non-compliance with these laws, and women's lack of knowledge of their rights and the power to demand them.

Consequently, statistics indicate that early breastfeeding (BF) cessation is associated with women's return to work, so it is of utmost importance to disseminate and provide a private and hygienic space, other than a bathroom, that women can use for expressing milk during their working day. It is therefore necessary to encourage companies to commit themselves to complying with the rules and laws. [3]

It is also well known that providing breastfeeding time for working women is one of the most important policies to facilitate women's continued ability to breastfeed. It also benefits companies by reducing absenteeism of working mothers due to less illness in children, less expenditure on medication and hospitalisation, and women in better health.

Breastfeeding and return to work

When the gestation period is over, it is always a longing to meet the newborn, to feel and look at the little fruit that one has been waiting so patiently for 9 months. These are once in a lifetime moments that one wants to enjoy to the full, but when the woman has a working life, returning to it can be a nightmare, the worry of leaving her little one can be frightening, frustrating and sad, especially when the mother has considered exclusive breastfeeding.

When mothers have to separate from their baby, the baby can continue to be breastfed. To do this, the mother will have to express the milk using an appropriate technique. The first thing to do is hand hygiene; if you are going to express manually, you should promote the ejection of the milk by massaging and rubbing the breast; then express the milk with movements that imitate the baby's sucking by pushing back and forth with your fingers about 3-4 centimetres behind the nipple. If you have a manual or electric breast pump, use it according to the manufacturer's recommendations, always maintaining the hygiene and sterilisation measures of the equipment. The milk should be expressed in clean and sterile plastic (Bisphenol A-BPA free) or glass containers.[2][4][6]

For storage, milk should be labelled with date and time of extraction and the conditions indicated should be observed. Frozen milk can be thawed in the refrigerator or by placing it in a container of water (water bath) but never directly exposed to flame or heated in a microwave oven. Thawed milk should not be refrozen and should be used as soon as possible.

Freezing periods for breast milk[4] .

Temperature.	Duration.
Environment:	6-8 hours
Refrigeration 4 to 8 °C	24 hours
Refrigerator (stored at the back)	5 days
Freezer separate from the chiller	3-6 months
Independent freezer	6-12 months

Steps to successful breastfeeding.

One of the main questions that many women ask themselves during the gestation process, mainly women who will be new mothers, is whether they will really be able to breastfeed their child properly. In this sense, when talking about this topic, sometimes women with previous experience can mention that other women who have already breastfed advise and describe that the attachment of the baby to the breast occurs naturally, as well as the baby's adaptation.

It is therefore important for the mother to consider that the mother-child bond is an individual experience, so she should not worry if it does not appear immediately. In the same sense, it takes time to get to know the newborn and the bond will be developed and strengthened by caring for the newborn. However, when the mother has to return to her place of work where she has to keep a work schedule, this process is complicated as the time allocated for breastfeeding is affected as there is not enough time for the baby. [6]

In this regard, the Federal Labour Law currently protects labour rights during pregnancy and breastfeeding, according to Articles 166, 167 and 170 of this law, during breastfeeding for a period of up to six months, there is the right to two breaks per day of half an hour each to feed the baby, in a place designated by the company with adequate hygienic conditions. In some situations this right for some women may not be enough to achieve successful breastfeeding, some mothers opt for other alternatives, preferring the extraction and freezing of breast milk so that the caregiver responsible for the newborn can provide feeding in the absence of the mother.[2]

For successful breastfeeding, new mothers need the support of the professionals who care for them during the first days of their baby's life, both in the maternity ward and in the health centre. Fortunately, hospitals are increasingly supportive of breastfeeding. In April 2018, the World Health Organization (WHO) and UNICEF updated their "Guidelines for the protection, promotion and support of breastfeeding in hospitals and health centres", which include steps for successful breastfeeding, i.e. the WHO's 10 tips on breastfeeding, so that health workers can support women before and after their gestational stage to feed their children correctly and effectively:

1. To have an institutional policy in favour of comprehensive care for mothers and children.
2. Train all health personnel on how to implement this policy.

3. Train pregnant women and their families in all aspects of breastfeeding.

4. Initiate breastfeeding within half an hour of birth.

5. Teaching mothers techniques and how to maintain breastfeeding.

6. Exclusively breastfeed newborns, only offering other types of food when medically indicated.

7. Facilitate and encourage co-housing.

8. Encourage breastfeeding on demand.

9. Do not give children bottles or dummies.

10. Encourage the establishment of support groups

Access to breastfeeding and adequate nutrition is a fundamental human right and the first measure of food security for a baby, which is why there are laws and recommendations that clearly define the best way to carry out and support breastfeeding outside and within companies. Therefore, for a mother returning to work after maternity leave should not be a reason to abandon breastfeeding, let alone risk losing her job.

It has been observed that sometimes it is not easy to combine breastfeeding with the demands of work; there are occasions when companies do not offer support for women who are breastfeeding, because they do not offer them the same opportunities for professional growth, which is the reason for the decrease in work productivity.

Allow breastfeeding women to take breaks and have flexible schedules to breastfeed their children or express their milk, and to store it in a suitable space such as a lactation room. This is a win-win situation: productive and motivated human talent, well-fed and healthy children, as well as a responsible and committed company.

When we hear about a breastfeeding room at work, our imagination runs wild, we start to think about what a place with breastfeeding women would be like in a company during working hours, especially in which area of the company a breastfeeding room would be installed. A breastfeeding room should be designated in a specific, dignified, private, hygienic and easily accessible area for all women who are breastfeeding or who express breast milk in order to provide a satisfactory continuity of breastfeeding.

Before designating an area for breastfeeding, the first step is to choose the area to be designated, taking into account the number of women of childbearing age and the conditions of space in the company.

Prior to the installation of a breastfeeding room in the work environment it is important to build a favourable environment that promotes a breastfeeding culture in the workplace and it is therefore recommended: [4]

- Make a formal commitment to breastfeeding among the company's management and staff.
- Receive training in breastfeeding techniques directly from a breastfeeding expert.
- Manage a breastfeeding room with the necessary supplies and policies for its proper functioning.

Model of a breastfeeding room.

The installation of a lactation room does not imply expenses that are economically damaging to a company, it really only implies a good organisation since it is not necessary to build a new place, it is only necessary to choose a space that meets the appropriate characteristics and to fit it out so that it can function as a lactation room. [4]

Once the company has a breastfeeding policy in place, the following steps are suggested for the proper functioning of the breastfeeding room.

1. The area designated for the breastfeeding room should be an accessible space that provides privacy and comfort for breastfeeding women workers.
2. Provide the equipment and material necessary for its proper functioning.
3. Assign a trained person to coordinate and manage the room.

4. Apply safety and hygiene standards to ensure the quality and preservation of breastmilk in the expression process.

Participants in a breastfeeding room.

Implementing and coordinating a breastfeeding room is not an easy task and requires the joint efforts of different partners to ensure that breastfeeding is not interrupted.

First of all, the human resources staff, through the person responsible for health or the person designated as responsible for the breastfeeding room, should inform the working woman of her rights during the breastfeeding stage and, together with the staff, provide a better working environment.

The person in charge of the breastfeeding room will have to fulfil various tasks which include disseminating the existence of the breastfeeding room among the staff, promoting the proper use of this space, as well as coordinating and verifying its proper maintenance and operation, and finally, making proposals for continuous improvement. [4]

Regulations for the use of the breastfeeding room.

It is important to have structured rules to ensure the correct use of the breastfeeding room, including the following:

1. Establish a timetable which will be determined by the number of users, breastfeeding schedules, the authorisation of the management of the work centre must be obtained, as the use of the room is exclusively for breastfeeding women.

2. Every woman who uses the room must sign in at each visit and must wash her hands when entering and leaving the room.

3. The use, cleaning and sterilisation of all equipment used during the visit in the lactation room is the responsibility of each client.

4. The lactation room is for breastfeeding or breast milk expression purposes only, and shall not be used for other purposes.

Conclusions

Analysing the bibliographic information that lists the multiple benefits of breastfeeding in women and newborns, not only at a physiological level, but also in an economic, social and emotional panorama, it is of utmost importance to offer more education and promotion programmes on breastfeeding, beyond being a talk given to working mothers, it should also include information for companies and business leaders, informing them about the laws and sanctions to which they may be subject if their labour rights are infringed.

It is recommended to analyse existing programmes and assess areas of opportunity in order to take appropriate action.

The World Health Organization, in conjunction with UNICEF, states that:

"The primary obligation of governments is to formulate, implement, monitor and evaluate a comprehensive national policy on infant and young child feeding. For such a policy to succeed, in addition to political commitment at the highest level, effective national coordination is required to ensure the full collaboration of all government agencies, international organizations and other stakeholders. To this end, information on food policies and practices needs to be collected and evaluated on an ongoing basis. Regional and local governments also have an important role to play in the implementation of this strategy."

References

Pan American Health Organization. World Breastfeeding Week 2020 - PAHO/WHO [Internet]. Paho.org. 2020 [cited 2022 Jun 17]. Available from: https://www.paho.org/es/campanas/semana-mundial-lactancia-materna-2020#:~:text=Breastfeeding%20is%20the%20mortality%20due%20to%20infectious%20diseases.

2. Sanchez I. Rights of Working Mothers in Mexico. Pregnancy, breastfeeding and childcare. [Internet]. Legalario. 2019 [cited 2022 Jun 17]. Available from: https://www.legalario.com/blog/derechos-de-las-madres-trabajadoras-en-mexico/#:~:text=Within%20the%20rights%20of,hygienic%20that%20the%20company%20designates.

Save the Children. The importance of breastmilk. [Internet]. 2021 [cited 2022 Jun 17]. Available from: https://blog.savethechildren.mx/2021/07/19/la-importancia-de-la-leche-materna/

4. Ministry of Labour and Social Security. Guide for the installation and operation of breastfeeding rooms [Internet]. Available from: https://www.gob.mx/cms/uploads/attachment/file/613760/Guia_de_Lactancia_Materna_en_el_Lugar_de_Trabajo.pdf

5. González T, Cordero S. Breastfeeding in Mexico [Internet]. Available from: https://www.anmm.org.mx/documentos-postura/LACTANCIA_MATERNA.pdf

6 . Ortega M. Recommendations for successful breastfeeding. Acta pediatr. Mex, Mexico. Vol. 3 (2). Pg. 126-129. (2015). Available at <http://www.scielo.org.mx/scielo.php?script=sci_arttext&pid=S0186-23912015000200011&lng=es&nrm=iso>. accessed 13 Dec. 2022.

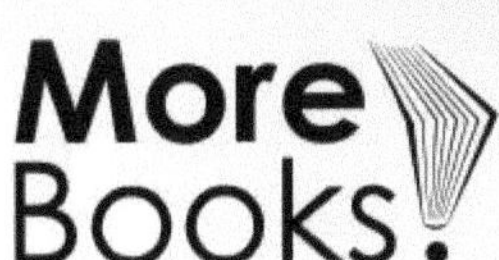

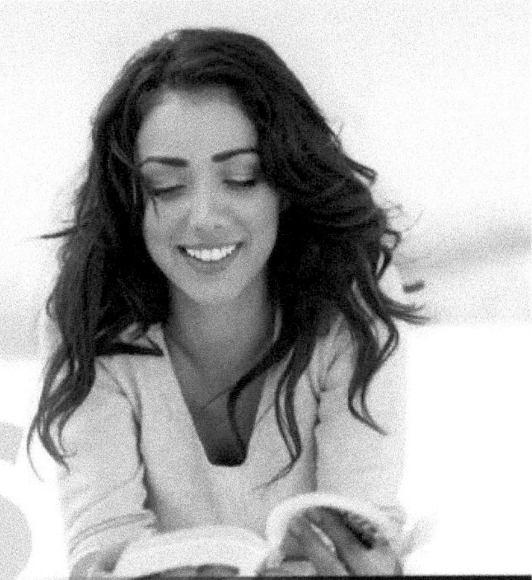

Buy your books fast and straightforward online - at one of world's fastest growing online book stores! Environmentally sound due to Print-on-Demand technologies.

Buy your books online at
www.morebooks.shop

Kaufen Sie Ihre Bücher schnell und unkompliziert online – auf einer der am schnellsten wachsenden Buchhandelsplattformen weltweit! Dank Print-On-Demand umwelt- und ressourcenschonend produzi ert.

Bücher schneller online kaufen
www.morebooks.shop

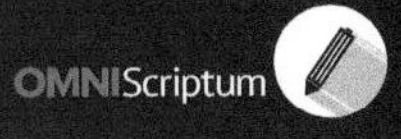

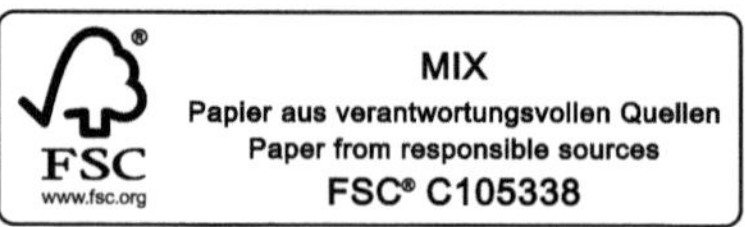

Printed by Books on Demand GmbH, Norderstedt / Germany